Number 103
Fall 2004

New Directions for Evaluation

Jean A. King
Editor-in-Chief

Ruth A. Bowan
Assistant Editor

Robin Miller
Katherine Ryan
Nancy Zajano
Associate Editors

Global Advances in HIV/AIDS Monitoring and Evaluation

T0220087

Deborah Rugg
Greet Peersman
Michel Carael
Editors

GLOBAL ADVANCES IN HIV/AIDS MONITORING AND EVALUATION
Deborah Rugg, Greet Peersman, Michel Carael (eds.)
New Directions for Evaluation, no. 103
Jean A. King, Editor-in-Chief
Copyright ©2004 Wiley Periodicals, Inc., A Wiley company

Microfilm copies of issues and articles are available in 16mm and 35mm, as well as microfiche in 105mm, through University Microfilms Inc., 300 North Zeeb Road, Ann Arbor, Michigan 48106-1346.

New Directions for Evaluation is indexed in Contents Pages in Education, Higher Education Abstracts, and Sociological Abstracts.

NEW DIRECTIONS FOR EVALUATION (ISSN 1097-6736, electronic ISSN 1534-875X) is part of The Jossey-Bass Education Series and is published quarterly by Wiley Subscription Services, Inc., a Wiley company, at Jossey-Bass, 989 Market Street, San Francisco, California 94103-1741.

SUBSCRIPTIONS cost $80.00 for U.S./Canada/Mexico; $104 international. For institutions, agencies, and libraries, $175 U.S.; $215 Canada; $249 international. Prices subject to change.

EDITORIAL CORRESPONDENCE should be addressed to the Editor-in-Chief, Jean A. King, University of Minnesota, 330 Wulling Hall, 86 Pleasant Street SE, Minneapolis, MN 55455.

www.josseybass.com

Editorial Policy and Procedures

New Directions for Evaluation, a quarterly sourcebook, is an official publication of the American Evaluation Association. The journal publishes empirical, methodological, and theoretical works on all aspects of evaluation. A reflective approach to evaluation is an essential strand to be woven through every volume. The editors encourage volumes that have one of three foci: (1) craft volumes that present approaches, methods, or techniques that can be applied in evaluation practice, such as the use of templates, case studies, or survey research; (2) professional issue volumes that present issues of import for the field of evaluation, such as utilization of evaluation or locus of evaluation capacity; (3) societal issue volumes that draw out the implications of intellectual, social, or cultural developments for the field of evaluation, such as the women's movement, communitarianism, or multiculturalism. A wide range of substantive domains is appropriate for *New Directions for Evaluation;* however, the domains must be of interest to a large audience within the field of evaluation. We encourage a diversity of perspectives and experiences within each volume, as well as creative bridges between evaluation and other sectors of our collective lives.

The editors do not consider or publish unsolicited single manuscripts. Each issue of the journal is devoted to a single topic, with contributions solicited, organized, reviewed, and edited by a guest editor. Issues may take any of several forms, such as a series of related chapters, a debate, or a long article followed by brief critical commentaries. In all cases, the proposals must follow a specific format, which can be obtained from the editor-in-chief. These proposals are sent to members of the editorial board and to relevant substantive experts for peer review. The process may result in acceptance, a recommendation to revise and resubmit, or rejection. However, the editors are committed to working constructively with potential guest editors to help them develop acceptable proposals.

Jean A. King, Editor-in-Chief
University of Minnesota
330 Wulling Hall
86 Pleasant Street SE
Minneapolis, MN 55455
e-mail: kingx004@umn.edu

CONTENTS

EDITORS' NOTES

The focus of this issue of *New Directions for Evaluation* is on global advances in monitoring and evaluation (M&E) of the global response to the human immunodeficiency virus-acquired immunodeficiency syndrome (HIV/AIDS) epidemic. The primary focus is on developing nations and is largely from the perspective of evaluators working for donors, international agencies, and national governments. Only by implementing comprehensive and sustainable M&E systems will we know how much progress we are making, as nations and as a global community, in combating this pandemic. The need for solid information on what is and is not working in real-life settings has never been stronger. HIV/AIDS M&E is currently receiving a lot of attention at the highest levels and in many international forums within the context of global health and security issues. Recent meetings include, for example, the G8 discussions that took place on Sea Island, Georgia (U.S.A) (G8, 2004) and the Conference on Scaling Up the Health Response to AIDS, Tuberculosis, and Malaria in Wilton Park, Great Britain (Institute for Global Health), both in June 2004. Evaluators who do not work in the field of HIV/ AIDS will also find the topics discussed of interest. Not only is the HIV/AIDS epidemic the largest public health disaster in almost one hundred years, the challenges faced and methods used are applications of mainstream evaluation, and by pushing the envelope the contributors have highlighted some of the limitations of current evaluation practice. As such, these discussions merit attention by evaluators in general and have relevance to other social and health problems, especially those that are highly complex, dynamic, and have large social and political implications.

Infectious diseases, old and new, and the multiple sources of funding to combat them, along with enhanced availability of treatments, have made M&E of HIV/AIDS prevention and treatment programs more complex and demanding than ever before. For example, the Global Fund to Fight AIDS, Tuberculosis and Malaria is one of the several new global initiatives targeting the strengthening of developing countries' response to HIV/AIDS and two other significant infectious diseases, namely tuberculosis and malaria. Newly developed country coordinating committees have been superimposed on already-existing national AIDS programs and national AIDS councils to coordinate the application of these funds for program implementation. The basic goal of this global funding initiative is, to use the often-cited phrase, "Raise it, spend it, prove it" (Global Fund to Fight AIDS, Tuberculosis and Malaria, 2004a). It is the global effort to "prove it" that is the focus of this issue. Whereas it has taken two decades to mobilize significant global resources to fight HIV/AIDS ("raise it"), the challenge is now to "spend it" effectively by implementing the right programs in a coordinated manner. The only way to know that this is indeed happening ("prove it") is by implementing effective, sustainable, and coordinated M&E systems that track resources, monitor progress, and evaluate program effectiveness.

If global goals for disease control are to be achieved, new and existing donors need to coordinate their assistance to developing countries by bringing together funding, planning, management, and reporting systems (Brugha and others, 2004). A joint and coordinated response to strengthen overall M&E capacity and health management information systems in developing nations is more likely to be effective than each agency tackling these issues separately for each separate disease. Many approaches to M&E can be shared across diseases, especially in resource-constrained settings where it is vital that duplication of effort and waste of resources be avoided. A common understanding of M&E language, frameworks, and methods is needed to facilitate sharing of information and true collaboration and coordination. We start the introduction to this issue with a discussion of the M&E language, guiding themes, and organizing framework within which the chapters' issues are presented. Subsequently, we provide an overview of how each of the chapters contributes to the discussion.

Harmonizing M&E Basics

The basics of effective HIV/AIDS M&E are a common language, guiding themes, and organizing frameworks.

Common Language

Agencies or individuals often use M&E terms interchangeably or in idiosyncratic ways. This inconsistent use of terms is particularly confusing as experts and lay managers develop and use guidance documents, implement joint M&E plans, and communicate across agencies and disciplines involved in M&E. Establishing a common language, therefore, should help to clarify meanings, identify specialized usages of terms in the HIV/AIDS arena, and foster a better overall understanding of M&E between experts and lay contributors alike. Because it is hoped that this issue will receive wide distribution beyond the general evaluation audience to program managers and policymakers involved in HIV/AIDS worldwide, definitions of relevant concepts as applied to global HIV/AIDS M&E are included in a glossary at the end of the Editors' Notes.

Guiding Themes and Organizing Frameworks

We offer three steps to planning and implementing an M&E strategy:

1. *Use a program-improvement, utilization-focused approach to collecting M&E data.* The first and perhaps the most important guiding theme for all M&E efforts is that information should be collected with the intention

of being used by key stakeholders, program managers, and policymakers for program improvement (Patton, 1997). Although reporting and accountability remain a priority for funding agencies, they have endorsed this basic M&E utilization focus. In principle, donors and multilateral agencies support a unified approach to strengthening the government and other stakeholders' capacity to collect and use M&E data that address the country's priority needs. However, the execution of this principle can vary significantly by agency and by country.

A donor-driven, reactive approach to M&E has contributed to the fragmentation of M&E efforts in many countries, creating one of the largest challenges facing HIV/AIDS M&E efforts today. The international M&E community has made some progress at the global headquarters levels by fostering partnerships and collaborative approaches among agencies such as the Joint United Nations Programme on HIV/AIDS (UNAIDS); the World Health Organization; the U.S. Agency for International Development; the U.S. Centers for Disease Control and Prevention; the World Bank; and the Global Fund to Fight AIDS, Tuberculosis and Malaria (Joint United Nations Programme on HIV/AIDS, 2000, and Global Fund to Fight AIDS, Tuberculosis and Malaria, 2004b). The next step is to focus on implementing a coordinated strategy at the country level.

2. *All M&E staff must serve as "catalysts for coordination" to foster coordination at all levels to minimize fragmentation and duplication of effort.* The second theme highlights the need for collaboration and coordination. Whereas the global focus in recent years has been on collaborative efforts to develop international M&E partnerships, standards, indicators, guidance documents, and collaborative networks, the present challenge is to foster coordination at the country level to decrease the fragmentation and redundancy referred to above. To address this, donor agencies at both headquarter and field offices are making several new attempts, including providing technical support for developing a single, national database; deploying additional M&E field staff; providing M&E training; increasing funding for M&E; and improving the harmonization of indicators and reporting requirements among donor agencies. These recent efforts have culminated in the endorsement by all major donor agencies and governments of the *Three Ones Principles: A Commitment to Concerted Action* (Joint United Nations Programme on HIV/AIDS, 2004). This commitment seeks to move the idea of a *single* national AIDS authority; a *single* national strategic plan; and a *single* comprehensive, strategic, and well-coordinated M&E system, into a reality.

3. *We must think strategically and have a road map.* The third guiding theme relates to the need to take a strategic and phased approach in the implementation of a comprehensive M&E system, acknowledging two realities: appropriate infrastructure and capacity must be in place to implement the different components of a comprehensive system—not everything can be done at once; and every program does *not* need to conduct all aspects of

Figure A. Strategic Planning for Monitoring and Evaluation: Setting Realistic Expectations

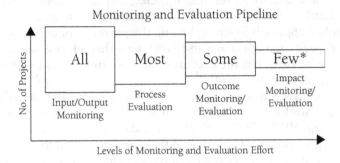

Monitoring and Evaluation Pipeline

No. of Projects

| All | Most | Some | Few* |

Input/Output Monitoring

Process Evaluation

Outcome Monitoring/ Evaluation

Impact Monitoring/ Evaluation

Levels of Monitoring and Evaluation Effort

Note: An asterisk indicates that this is supplemented with impact indicators from surveillance data.

M&E. A frequently used diagram to explain the latter is the "M&E pipeline" shown in Figure A (Rugg and Mills, 2000).

This M&E pipeline is based on the simple *input-activities-outputs-outcomes-impact* framework that most agencies now endorse (see Chapter Two, this issue). This diagram suggests that *all programs* should conduct basic program input and output monitoring for the purposes of good program management and for selecting a few indicators (for example, number of people tested, number of clients served, number of people trained, or number of condoms distributed) to report to key stakeholders to whom the program is accountable. *Most programs* should also conduct some basic process evaluations. This component often includes implementation assessments, quality assessments, basic operations research, case studies, and cost analyses. Only *some* programs will be able to conduct outcome monitoring and even fewer rigorous outcome evaluations, not only because of the additional time, expertise, and resources that these methods require but also because they are only relevant to the more established programs (outcome monitoring) or programs for which there is insufficient evidence that they work (outcome evaluation).

Finally, only in *few* cases would impact evaluation be warranted in which an attempt is made to attribute long-term effects (impact) to a specific program. However, monitoring the unlinked distal impacts (impact monitoring) can feasibly be done through surveillance systems and repeated population-based biological and behavioral surveys (see Chapter Two, this issue). All programs should be aware of these national and subnational data and how these are relevant to their program. They typically provide a basis for comparing national and local program output and outcome monitoring efforts. In other words, in determining the overall success or collective effectiveness of all programs that constitute the national response to HIV/AIDS, it is necessary to interpret long-term effects in the context of results from process and outcome evaluations and from existing survey data and output monitoring. The main strategic point here is simple: Not everybody needs to do everything!

The M&E pipeline diagram is only one way to help conceptualize a basic M&E approach. Other diagrams are described in Chapter Two. Together they provide the historical and conceptual basis for organizing our approach to HIV/AIDS M&E in general.

The basic building blocks and strategy for implementing a national M&E system, then, are the following:

- A strategic questions approach for setting priorities, with participation by all stakeholders
- A comprehensive national strategic M&E plan, addressing both monitoring and evaluation needs and including adequate resources
- A realistic work plan, with a phased implementation approach
- Strategic, coordinated implementation with sound M&E management, adequately trained staff, and sustainable technical assistance to support the entire system.

Current Status of M&E

Whereas a comprehensive M&E system must eventually include both monitoring and evaluation activities to fully track the epidemic, target and inform the response, design better programs, and understand what is and is not working, the initial focus of the global response has been to establish a foundation derived largely from surveys and monitoring information. It is no surprise, therefore, that the chapters in this issue—and, indeed, the overall literature in this area—focus mainly on survey and monitoring efforts, as depicted in Figure B. This diagram suggests that two aspects need to be examined and can be used to measure our progress toward implementing comprehensive M&E: the ability to make causal inferences and the utility of the data for program improvement. The first regards the ability to make causal inferences about a program's consequences, with simple monitoring by itself affording little ability to make such inferences. As monitoring data from multiple sources are triangulated and supplemented with appropriate evaluation designs, logical plausibility and causality are strengthened. The second regards the utility of the data acquired for program improvement. Here accountability data often afford the least amount of information relevant to program improvement and need to be supplemented by relevant program information and appropriate evaluation designs. This depiction of the current status of HIV/AIDS M&E shows that we have a long way to go toward having both sufficient monitoring and essential evaluations.

Given the limited resources that have been available for M&E in general and for rigorous evaluations in particular, the initial overall focus on

Figure B. Status of HIV/AIDS Program Monitoring and Evaluation

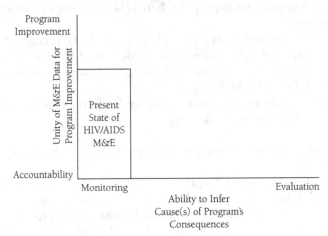

monitoring was appropriate. However, this situation is now changing because more funding for M&E efforts is available, and our understanding of what is needed is now more sophisticated.

Introduction to This Issue

Given the urgency of the global response to the AIDS epidemic, we felt it timely to present a series of articles devoted to global HIV/AIDS M&E. The chapters are grouped by the level they are representing: that is, global-level or donor perspectives; country-level or national perspectives; and project-level or program perspectives. To date, much of the focus in M&E has come from the global level as many new global funding initiatives have been launched and required rapid scaling up and the development of technical guidance, international standards, and indicators for monitoring progress and determining success. The first five chapters reflect this global or donor perspective. The subsequent three chapters describe regional and country-level perspectives, and the final chapter before the commentaries describes the status of project-level intervention research and targeted program evaluations.

We begin with a look at the global developments in HIV/AIDS M&E and the context in which these have occurred. In Chapter One, Paul De Lay and Valerie Manda discuss the political issues surrounding the global response to HIV/AIDS, and Deborah Rugg, Michel Carael, Ties Boerma, and John Novak provide in Chapter Two an overview of the history of AIDS M&E, from the initial case reporting of AIDS to complex surveillance activities and the development of M&E frameworks.

Next, a critical look is taken at the role of key agencies in advancing the global agenda for HIV/AIDS M&E. In Chapter Three, Nicole Massoud, Paul De Lay, and Michel Carael discuss UNAIDS and its role in developing core standardized international indicators to monitor the Declaration of Commitment on HIV/AIDS, which was signed by 189 member nations at the United Nations General Assembly Special Session on HIV/AIDS held in June 2001 (United Nations General Assembly Special Session on HIV/AIDS, 2001). The process used to develop these indicators and the lessons learned from the first progress report are the substance of this chapter. Next, global interagency collaboration and in-country coordination are examined in Chapter Four (by Deborah Rugg and others) that describes the experiences of two U.S government agencies—the U.S. Agency for International Development and the U.S. Centers for Disease Control and Prevention. The authors take an in-depth look at interagency collaboration at the global and national levels and highlight lessons learned from both the headquarters and field perspectives, providing an example from Cambodia.

Because therapy for HIV/AIDS is rapidly becoming available to many developing nations, Cameron Wolf and others (Chapter Five) take a special look at global efforts to develop and field test monitoring indicators for the expanded care and treatment programs for HIV/AIDS. The authors examine the challenges faced in monitoring these efforts, along with results from the first field tests jointly supported by the World Health Organization and others.

The issue then shifts focus from the global-level to the regional and country-level perspective. David Wilson in Chapter Six assesses the capacity of national governments in southern Africa to conduct M&E activities and critically examines the World Bank's support for M&E capacity-building efforts at the country level. In Chapter Seven, Siripon Kanshana and others present an example of a successful national M&E system to monitor the National Program to Prevent Mother-to-Child Transmission of HIV in Thailand. This chapter is followed by an in-depth look in Chapter Eight at the establishment of a national M&E system in Ghana, a country with extensive decentralization. Sylvia Anie and Emmanuel Larbi discuss the lessons learned in implementing a participatory approach to this process.

Finally, based on an extensive systematic literature review, Greet Peersman and Deborah Rugg (Chapter Nine) focus on the project-level perspective and discuss the paucity of evaluation studies in general and the lack of rigorous evaluations in particular. Without adequate evaluations, there is no measure of how effective or ineffective interventions are, which hinders decision making regarding the scaling up of interventions.

The issue concludes with two commentaries written in response to the articles. Nicolas Meda, an evaluation epidemiologist in Burkina Faso in West Africa, highlights in Chapter Ten the difficulties developing countries face in responding to global expectations for HIV/AIDS M&E. His commentary serves as a voice from the field as he reflects on the relevance of the M&E approaches discussed in this issue. He provides valuable insight into the needs and concerns of both developing country governments and organizations working in these countries. Michael Quinn Patton, an international evaluation consultant, then provides a broader view in Chapter Eleven, linking the evaluation problems and issues discussed in this journal with those from other areas of evaluation. He comments on whether global HIV/AIDS M&E can serve as a prototype for other areas of M&E and challenges us all to consider alternative evaluation methods, to remember to include the voices of those affected, and to move rapidly beyond collecting monitoring indicators only.

We thank the reviewers for their assistance in making this a stronger issue; for example, Figure B was based on insightful feedback from an early reviewer. We also acknowledge the valuable contribution to this issue by Anne Stangl, a graduate student at Tulane University, New Orleans, who served as the issue coordinator and editorial assistant. She provided outstanding assistance in organizing the process, interacting with the authors, and keeping things on track.

References

Brugha, R., and others. "The Global Fund: Managing Great Expectations." *Lancet*, 2004, *364*, 95–100.

Centers for Disease Control and Prevention. *Monitoring and Evaluation Capacity Building for Program Improvement. Field Guide.* (Version 1.) Atlanta: Global AIDS Program, Centers for Disease Control and Prevention, 2003.

G8. *Chair's Statement.* 2004. [http://www.g8usa.gov/d_061004m.htm]. Retrieved June 23, 2004.

Global Fund to Fight AIDS, Tuberculosis and Malaria. *The Framework Document of The Global Fund to Fight AIDS, Tuberculosis and Malaria.* Geneva: Global Fund to Fight AIDS, Tuberculosis and Malaria, 2000.

Global Fund to Fight AIDS, Tuberculosis and Malaria. *Annual Report 2003.* Geneva: Global Fund to Fight AIDS, Tuberculosis and Malaria, 2004a.

Global Fund to Fight AIDS, Tuberculosis and Malaria. *Monitoring and Evaluation Toolkit.* Geneva: Global Fund to Fight AIDS, Tuberculosis and Malaria, 2004b.

Institute for Global Health. *Conference Proceedings: Scaling Up the Health Response to AIDS, Tuberculosis, and Malaria.* San Francisco: University of California, San Francisco, 2004.

Joint United Nations Programme on HIV/AIDS. *National AIDS Programs: A Guide to Monitoring and Evaluation.* Geneva: Joint United Nations Programme on HIV/AIDS, 2000.

Joint United Nations Programme on HIV/AIDS. "'Three Ones' Key Principles: A Coordination of National Response to HIV/AIDS." Conference paper for Washington Consultation, Washington, D.C., Apr. 2004. [http://www.unaids.org/NetTools/Misc/DocInfo.aspx?href=http%3A%2F%2Fgva%2Ddoc%2Dowl%2FWEBcontent%2FDocuments%2Fpub%2FUNA%2Ddocs%2FThree%2DOnes%5FKeyPrinciples%5Fen%2Epdf]. Retrieved June 23, 2004.

Patton, M. Q. *Utilization-Focused Evaluation.* (3rd ed.) Thousand Oaks, Calif.: Sage, 1997.

Rugg, D., and Mills, S. "Development of an Integrated Monitoring and Evaluation Plan." In T. Rehle, T. Saidel, S. Mills, and R. Magnani (eds.), *Evaluating Programs for*

HIV/AIDS Prevention and Care in Developing Countries. Arlington, Va.: Family Health International, 2000.

United Nations General Assembly Special Session on HIV/AIDS. "The Declaration of Commitment on HIV/AIDS." 2001. [http://www.unaids.org]. Retrieved June 23, 2004.

Deborah Rugg
Greet Peersman
Michel Carael
Editors

Glossary of Selected Monitoring and Evaluation Terms

Antiretroviral therapy (ART) or antiretroviral (ARV). A medical treatment regimen that fights the human immunodeficiency virus (HIV) in those diagnosed with acquired immunodeficiency syndrome (AIDS)

Baseline. The status of services and outcome-related measures such as knowledge, attitudes, norms, behaviors, and conditions before an intervention.

Case study. A methodological approach to describing a situation, individual, or the like that typically incorporates data-gathering activities—interviews, observations, questionnaires—at selected sites or programs; the findings are then used to report to stakeholders, make recommendations for program improvement, and share lessons with other countries

Coverage. The extent to which a program reaches its intended target population, institution, or geographical area

Disease surveillance. The ongoing systematic collection, analysis, and interpretation of data to describe diseases and their transmission in populations; these data can help predict future trends and target needed prevention and treatment programs; when the data are collected from certain sites—hospitals, antenatal clinics—that are believed to be representative of the population and have the potential to serve as early warning signs (sentinels), the process is called *sentinel surveillance*

Evaluation. A rigorous, scientifically based collection of information about program activities, characteristics, and outcomes that determine the merit or worth of a specific program; evaluation studies are used to improve programs and inform decisions about future resource allocations

Facility survey. A site inventory of all elements required to deliver services, such as basic infrastructure, drugs, equipment, test kits, registers, and staff trained in the delivery of the service; the units of observation are facilities of various types and levels in the health system and normally include both public and private facilities in the sample frame of sites; may also be referred to as a *service provision assessment*

Impact. The longer-range, cumulative effect of programs over time, such as change in HIV infection, morbidity, and mortality; impacts are rarely, if ever, attributable to a single program, but a program may, with other programs, contribute to impacts on a population

Impact evaluation. Looks at the rise and fall of disease incidence and prevalence as a function of HIV/AIDS programs; the effects (impact) on entire populations seldom can be attributed to a single program or even several programs; therefore, evaluations of impact on populations usually entail a rigorous evaluation design that includes the combined effects of a number of programs on at-risk populations

Impact monitoring. In the field of public health, is usually referred to as *disease surveillance* (see above) and is concerned with the monitoring of disease prevalence or incidence; with this type of monitoring, data are collected at the jurisdictional, regional, and national levels

Input. A resource used in a program; includes monetary and personnel resources that come from a variety of sources, as well as curricula and materials

Input and output monitoring. Involves the basic tracking of information about program inputs, or resources that go into a program, and about outputs of the program activities; data sources for monitoring inputs and outputs usually exist naturally in program documentation, such as activity reports and logs, and client records, which offer details about the time, place, and amount of services delivered, as well as the types of clients receiving services

Management information system (MIS). A data system, usually computerized, that routinely collects and reports information about the delivery of services, costs, demographical and health information, and results status

Monitoring and evaluation (M&E) plan. A comprehensive planning document for all M&E activities, it documents the key M&E questions to be addressed, what indicators are collected, how, how often, from where and why they will be collected; baselines, targets and assumptions; how they are going to be analyzed or interpreted, and how or how often reports will be developed and distributed on these indicators

Monitoring. The routine tracking and reporting of priority information about a program and its intended outputs and outcomes

National-level reports. Various sources of information that are used to describe program inputs and program-related, project-level activities countrywide; examples include reports of nongovernmental agencies and national reports on program progress, performance, strategies, and plans

Objective. A statement of desired, specific, realistic, and measurable program results

Operations research. Applies systematic research techniques to improve service delivery; this type of research and evaluation analyzes only factors that are under the control of program managers, such as improving the quality of services, increasing training and supervision of staff, and adding new service components; it is designed to assess the accessibility, availability, quality, and sustainability of programs

Outcome. The effect of program activities on target audiences or populations, such as change in knowledge, attitudes, beliefs, skills, behaviors, access to services, policies, and environmental conditions

Outcome evaluation. A type of evaluation that is concerned with determining if, and by how much, program activities or services achieved their intended outcomes; whereas outcome monitoring is helpful and necessary in knowing whether outcomes were attained, outcome evaluation attempts to attribute observed change to the intervention tested, describe the extent or scope of program outcomes, and indicate what might happen in the absence of the program; it is methodologically rigorous and requires a comparative element in design, such as a control or comparison group

Outcome monitoring. The basic tracking of variables that have been adopted as measures or "indicators" of the desired program outcomes; with national AIDS programs, it is typically conducted through population-based surveys to track whether desired outcomes have been reached; it may also track information directly related to program clients, such as change in knowledge, attitudes, beliefs, skills, behaviors, access to services, policies, and environmental conditions

Output. The results of program activities; relates to the direct products or deliverables of program activities, such as number of counseling sessions completed, number of people reached, and number of materials distributed

Population-based surveys. A large-scale national health survey, such as the Demographic and Health Survey

Process evaluation. Type of evaluation that focuses on program implementation, adding a dimension to the information that was tracked in input and output monitoring; usually focuses on a single program and uses largely qualitative methods to describe program activities and perceptions, especially during the developmental stages and early implementation of a program; may also include some quantitative approaches, such as surveys about client satisfaction and perceptions about needs and services; in addition, might provide understanding about a program's cultural, sociopolitical, legal, and economic contexts that affect programs

Program records. Various sources of information that are used to describe program inputs and program-related, project-level activities; examples include budget and expenditure records and logs of commodities

Reliability. Consistency and dependability of data collected through repeated use of a scientific instrument or data collection procedure used under the same conditions; is independent of data validity—that is, a data collection method may produce consistent data but not measure what is intended to be measured

Research. Focuses primarily on hypothesis testing in a controlled environment; it typically attempts to make statements about the relationships among specific variables under controlled circumstances and at a given point in time

Stakeholder. Person, group, or entity that has a role and interest in the goals or objectives and implementation of a program

Sustainability (of a program). Sufficient likelihood that political and financial support

Validity. The extent to which a measurement or test accurately measures what is intended to be measured

Source: Centers for Disease Control and Prevention, Global AIDS Program, Monitoring and Evaluation Team, 2003.

DEBORAH RUGG is the associate director of the Monitoring and Evaluation Team for the Global AIDS Program at the U.S. Centers for Disease Control and Prevention, Atlanta, Georgia.

GREET PEERSMAN is the technical deputy director of the Monitoring and Evaluation Team for the Global AIDS Program at the U.S. Centers for Disease Control and Prevention, Atlanta, Georgia.

MICHEL CARAEL retired from the chief evaluation position in the Joint United Nations Programme on HIV/AIDS in 2004 and is currently a professor at the Free University of Brussels, Belgium, and consultant in evaluation.

1

Monitoring and evaluation programs must strike a balance between generating meaningful tactical information for program managers while taking steps to ensure that public data use does not worsen discrimination and stigma toward people who are positive for the human immunodeficiency virus.

Politics of Monitoring and Evaluation: Lessons from the AIDS Epidemic

Paul De Lay, Valerie Manda

Conventional monitoring and evaluation (M&E) textbooks rarely address the various political influences exerted on M&E of public health programs. Policymakers are often the largest consumers of M&E information; indeed, the genesis of many public health program evaluation efforts is a need to inform public policy. We define *political influences,* however, as external pressures that may suppress, limit, delay, manipulate, or selectively use M&E outputs. Such forces alter the accuracy and comprehensiveness of assessments of public health problems while coloring our understanding of program progress or effectiveness (Fox, 1999). Political influences originate from diverse sources and manifest as singular voices or power coalitions including government, industry, religious groups, lobbyists, organized labor, scientists, and special-interest groups (Epstein, 1996). Another often-overlooked source of political influence comes from within the institutions being assessed or those that implement M&E activities.

The world of politics is one of value conflict, as Laswell's (1958) definition of politics makes clear; competing policies further different, but not mutually exclusive, goals. It is indeed rare to find situations where compromises are not required or possible. The interaction, then, between politics and monitoring is no different in this respect. These interactions are not static and vary over time based on culture, administrative turnover, and the relative power of special-interest groups.

In this chapter, we do not present the overarching politics of human immunodeficiency virus-acquired immunodeficiency syndrome (HIV/AIDS). Excellent comprehensive resources exist that address this issue (Parker, 2002; Zuger, 2003; Burkhalter, 2004). Rather, we concentrate on the effects of discrete political influences on M&E efforts dealing with the HIV/AIDS epidemic and the effectiveness of the response. This chapter focuses on the HIV/AIDS pandemic to illustrate how political influences have resulted in noteworthy misuses of data, limiting response and fueling both stigma and discrimination.

Unfortunately, the AIDS epidemic is not unique where data misuse is concerned. Innumerable other examples may be cited where data are politically misrepresented, delaying effective response. Political forces are sometimes counterproductive and touch the broader arenas of public interaction and public health (Editors of *Lancet*, 2004; Colmers and Fox, 2003; Schneider and Fassin, 2002; Durban Declaration, 2000; Fox, 1999; Epstein, 1996; Laswell, 1958). Examples include political manipulation of M&E activities assessing emotionally charged subjects (reproductive choice, rape, child abuse, family violence), polarizing forces (privatization and social services reform; racial, gender, and ethnic equity), and government accountability to citizens (policing, infrastructure, education, defense) (Blackburn, 2004; Human Rights Watch, 2003, 2004a, 2004b; Transparency International, 2004; United Nations Children's Fund, 2003a, 2003b; United Nations Development Fund, 2002). Recently, M&E scrutiny into public health responses mounted to identify and contain infectious diseases such as severe, acute respiratory syndrome (SARS), West Nile virus, bovine spongiform encephalitis (mad cow disease), and avian flu, to name a few, have been politicized by economic, ideological, and scientific stakeholders (Parry, 2004; Reilly and others, 2003; Abbasi, 2000; Lacey, 1994).

It is understandable that there is little formal, published documentation on this subject. An exhaustive search of the clinical, public health, foreign affairs, political, economics, and social sector literature reveals only a few relevant articles, many of which come from the developed world. These references are cited in this chapter, but much of what we discuss comes from our personal experiences, communications with key informants involved with the epidemic, and through comparison with other diseases that have similar characteristics to the AIDS pandemic (Joint United Nations Programme on HIV/AIDS, 2000).

The relationship between politics and M&E is not necessarily negative; examples in this chapter indicate where strong, courageous political decisions have significantly advanced the M&E agenda. The chapter ends with conclusions and possible recommendations on how some of these potential problems can be addressed. Four areas of political-M&E tension will be explored:

- Global denial: Do we have a problem?
- Data use conflict: accountability versus programmatic information
- Protection of individual rights versus the public good
- Selective application of evaluation research in support of ideologies and values

This is not intended to be an exhaustive account but represents some of the more common issues those engaged in HIV/AIDS M&E confront.

HIV/AIDS Pandemic

Rarely has containment of an infectious disease epidemic evoked such challenge to humanity as has the HIV pandemic (van Niekerk, 2001). The effects that HIV and AIDS exert on economies, the fabric of families and communities, civil society, religious beliefs, and political systems have been well described (Burkhalter, 2004; Debt, AIDS, Trade, Africa, 2004; United Nations Children's Fund, 2003b; Arndt and Lewis, 2000). At each stage of the disease process, obstacles complicate effective responses: absence of totally effective prevention interventions; stigma associated with the modes of transmission; the terminal nature of the disease, particularly in settings with limited testing and antiretroviral therapy access; and the lack of curative therapies. However, in coping with this pandemic, there may be reason for guarded optimism as more information is gathered, innovative ways of responding are recognized, and a more nuanced understanding of the political stakes underlying public health agendas is gained.

In the case of HIV/AIDS, its sexual and injection-drug use transmission routes morally color the picture, a tempting and convenient explanation for potentially negative political responses. In a survey of U.S. reproductive services offered in American schools, Wald, Button, and Rienzo found that "service levels were influenced not only by cultural considerations. . . . [morality politics] but also by the same socioeconomic forces that account for policy levels in other domains" (2001, p. 221). They conclude that "policy for morality issues appears different from that for non-morality issues but less distinctive than commonly imagined" (p. 221). Their findings lend support to diminishing our exceptionalist view of HIV/AIDS transmission politics.

Global Denial: Do We Have a Problem?

Sin, stigma, and denial have accompanied unexplained diseases throughout the ages. Historically, some of the most notorious examples illustrating institutional denial of impending epidemics are illustrated by city-state responses to the plagues that swept across Europe in the late thirteenth century (Scott and Duncan, 2001; Ziegler, 1991). Of note, a few of these governments were relatively transparent about the effects of the plague, despite serious threats of economic disaster and quarantine. This may have occurred because the exact cause and modes of plague transmission were poorly understood. Further, many city-states were not powerful enough to prevent the dissemination of information beyond their boundaries. However, most denied the existence of plague infection within their jurisdictions. In Florence, more than one year after the plague was evident, the city's Great Council remained silent. "Perhaps the Councillors believed, not without reason, that it did not lie in their power to avert disaster and that, therefore, the less said the better" (Ziegler, 1991, p. 39).

Since the recognition of the first cases of HIV/AIDS in 1981, data on its prevalence have often been subject to official manipulation. Although relatively simple and inexpensive HIV testing methods exist and subpopulation seroprevalence data within countries should be relatively easy to obtain, national governments have continued to maintain secrecy on true prevalence and even deny the presence of HIV and AIDS. A variation on the denial of HIV infection prevalence is denial of it as the cause of AIDS. One of the most famous examples of this occurred in 2000 when South African President Thabo Mbeki wrote that he doubted HIV causes AIDS. This unleashed a firestorm of criticism from the scientific community; more than 5,000 scientists ultimately signed the subsequent Durban Declaration (2000) affirming that HIV causes AIDS. Others have argued that Mbeki was misquoted from the beginning and that his comments were meant to state that HIV *alone* is not the cause of AIDS, emphasizing the multifactorial nature of the epidemic. Poverty, for example, has been linked to exacerbation of HIV in the developing world (Debt, AIDS, Trade, Africa, 2004; Gow, 2002).

South Africa is not unique: in the early days of the epidemic, almost all countries in sub-Saharan Africa denied or diminished the extent of the problem. This was especially the case before a landmark meeting of the World Health Assembly in Geneva, Switzerland, in May 1987 and a subsequent meeting in London, England, of ministers of health in 1988 (Sabatier, 1988). Governments, anticipating public scrutiny and negative impact to their political authority, diminished or suppressed prevalence numbers, delayed reports, or implied that infected persons were primarily "foreign" (Sabatier, 1988). In fact, this has been more the rule than the exception, as both developing and developed countries confront a burgeoning epidemic.

Developed countries' municipal, provincial, and federal governments, particularly in the early part of the epidemic, often minimized threat to the overall population posed by HIV transmission by implying that the risk of infection was confined to "high-risk groups." This has resulted in the stubborn lingering popular opinion among average U.S. citizens that HIV risk is isolated to gay men and injection-drug users. This stereotype, perpetuated by overplayed early risk evaluation data coupled with persistent structural discrimination toward high-risk populations, presents an obstacle to prevention efforts. M&E data were used to assign risk to groups of people rather than to risky behaviors. Fortunately, such assignments have reversed. Risky behaviors, such as commercial sex work, injecting drugs, and unprotected sexual intercourse, contribute to the growing epidemic because of not only the risk presented to the individuals themselves but also the pathways and bridges they make, carrying HIV to their partners in the general population worldwide (Choi, Gibson, Han, and Guo, 2004). For this reason, partners who are not engaged in risky behavior themselves do not perceive themselves at risk of HIV infection, but they are still vulnerable.

Many reasons exist for such denial:

• Protection of a country's reputation and culture
• Embarrassment about discussing the prevalent modes of transmission, particularly when they conflict with dominant religious and cultural beliefs
• Perceived negative effects on tourism and economic investment
• Being forced to acknowledge the existence of marginalized or potentially "illegal" subpopulations (for example, men who have sex with men, commercial sex workers, and injection-drug users).

Interventions for these populations are sensitive, and access to strategic information from them is often restricted. Over the past two decades, governments have denied both the existence and extent of such so-called immoral behaviors. Stigma, discrimination, and exclusion often stem from inappropriate use of subpopulation epidemiological data (Poindexter, 2004; Stansbury and Sierra, 2004; Gow, 2002). In the United States and Latin America, where AIDS was first identified in the gay communities of New York, San Francisco, Washington, D.C., and Sao Paolo, Brazil, discrimination against same-sex intercourse undoubtedly fueled AIDS-related stigma. Also, in the United States in mid-1982, the Centers for Disease Control and Prevention (CDC) identified higher-than-expected infection rates among Haitian patients. Soon Haitian immigrants were included with other "high-risk" populations. It was not until three years later that the CDC focused on specific risk behaviors (men who have sex with men, tainted blood supply) as the root of increased prevalence, not nationality (Sabatier, 1988). Damage, however, had already been done, and in the early to mid-1980s, Haitian immigrants to the United States experienced employment discrimination while Haiti itself saw a dramatic drop in tourism (Sabatier, 1988).

Ever more frequently, national security interests and efforts to maintain a façade of civil stability are behind denial or manipulation of HIV prevalence statistics. On the African continent, perhaps the most urgent threat to security and stability is the AIDS crisis. African communities are losing the most able-bodied citizens who form the backbone of their civil societies: farmers, traditional leaders, teachers, doctors, nurses, soldiers, and law enforcement, to name a few (Cohen, 2002; Government of Malawi, 2002). Moreover, African families are losing their parents, leaving an entire generation of orphans to raise themselves (U.S. Agency for International Development, 2002). The onslaught of AIDS threatens to single-handedly undermine any economic progress made, actually leading to the expansion of poverty (Jamison, Sachs, and Wang, 2001; Arndt and Lewis, 2000). This makes the response to the AIDS pandemic one of paramount urgency and importance. Yet, an almost universal lack of openness has marred initial responses. Uganda, however, represents an admirable turnaround from the rampant global denial of the late 1980s.

The east African state of Uganda achieved independence from the United Kingdom in 1962. The infamous dictatorial regime of Idi Amin (1971 to 1979) was responsible for the deaths of some 300,000 opponents; guerrilla war and human rights abuses under Milton Obote (1980 to 1985) claimed at least another 100,000 lives. By 1986, political upheaval, horrific violence, and economic breakdown had crippled Uganda. The incoming government of President Yoweri Museveni—with the support of foreign countries and international aid agencies—needed to rehabilitate the country and stabilize the economy. At that moment, the AIDS epidemic erupted, and by early 1990, Uganda had become its African epicenter (U.S. Central Intelligence Agency, 2004).

Museveni, in dealing with the epidemic, has often acknowledged that his initial push came from Cuban President Fidel Castro during a meeting of the Non-Aligned Movement of developing countries in Harare, Zimbabwe, in September 1986. President Castro apparently called him and told him that eighteen of the sixty Ugandan soldiers who had been sent for training in Cuba had tested positive for HIV. This shocked Museveni into action. Despite a lack of cure or a vaccine, HIV infection rates are actually declining in Uganda. In 1991, 21 percent of pregnant women were HIV-positive; ten years later, that number declined to 6 percent. Uganda took an open, comprehensive, and courageous approach that has largely defused HIV stigma there. The heart of Uganda's approach has been behavioral change, promoted by the "ABC" model: Abstinence, Being faithful, and Condom use. As a result, in Uganda's heterosexually driven HIV epidemic, sexual activity among youth dropped and men reduced the number of sexual partners they had, contributing to this success story in AIDS response (Peterson, 2003).

In Asia, where the epidemic is relatively more recent than in Africa, we have seen the denial scenario repeated. In China, for instance, the ruling authority's tendency toward secrecy and the ensuing lack of public awareness have hampered HIV control efforts (Watts, 2003). Over the past two years, however, great progress has been shown in China's openness about the epidemic and an increased emphasis on the collection and dissemination of reliable epidemiological data. Some attribute this new transparency to the recent outbreaks of SARS. The first Asian SARS case was reported by Carlo Urbani from the World Health Organization (WHO) in February 2003 in Hanoi, Vietnam. Subsequent Chinese reporting delays concealed that SARS had actually been present in Asia well before 2003. The Vice Minister of Health in China eventually admitted that the initial Chinese response "had been slow and inadequate" (Drazen, 2003). With the second outbreak in 2004, however, Chinese officials ordered the slaughter of tens of thousands of mammals in a drastic measure to control the spread of a new SARS virus strain. The SARS epidemic showed that political will and international collaboration come together easily when only one country holds the key to solving questions crucial to global control of disease (Drazen, 2003).

Other factors may also influence the openness and dissemination of epidemiological data. Interestingly, coinciding with the influx of financial resources earmarked for AIDS from donors like the Global Fund to Fight AIDS, Tuberculosis and Malaria (Global Fund) and the World Bank Multicountry AIDS Program, some countries have upwardly revised their AIDS epidemic reporting. We are now witnessing, for example, a correlation between more timely and accurate reporting of HIV/AIDS prevalence and governmental perception that doing so will enhance access to these new financial resources. Of concern is potential embellishment of the prevalence trend, particularly among middle-income countries where proof of severity and burden of disease provide documentation necessary for obtaining significant new resources.

Monitoring Program Performance: Dominant Donor Needs

Strategic information that may be most useful to public health program managers is often asynchronous with the needs of international donors. Until recently, most international donors were actually sovereign governments, with significant funding coming from various U.S. agencies (U.S. Agency for International Development, CDC, State Department, and the like). Now, the Global Fund, the World Bank Multicountry AIDS Program, and private health and human rights philanthropy foundations (for example, the Bill and Melinda Gates Foundation, Open Society) have become more important in funding particular priority diseases.

Historically, M&E data have primarily served the accountability needs of the donor community. Indicators have focused on national outcome and impact data, rarely serving the daily practical decision-making needs of program managers. Statistics revealing district-level service use, patient satisfaction, and short-term clinical outcomes, although useful to program managers, often do not satisfy donor requirements to demonstrate national-level effects and financial accountability. Undoubtedly, donor countries and foundations must demonstrate the value of their investments to justify these expenditures and continue funding. This need has led to the rather common phenomenon that most existing M&E data for HIV/AIDS are generated through externally supported, designed, and implemented surveys, which are funded by the interested donor. Involvement of the national and subnational programs has been less than optimal.

An additional problem rooted in the role of donors as the primary users of strategic program information is an ongoing need for attribution: Whose money was responsible for which achievements? Program successes, however, typically result from multiple complementing activities. Yet, most donors still require data directly linking their financial investments in programs to improved or saved lives. This leads to laborious exercises where commodities and services are measured relative to a donor's input, often at the opportunity cost of other evaluation analyses that are more program-management related.

Increasingly, the tracking of financial resources is becoming a key component of basic M&E activities. The implementation of national health accounts (NHA) and national AIDS accounts (NAA) allows program decision makers to track where resources are flowing and whether they are being used in as effective a manner as possible. Through NHA and NAA, critical information may be obtained about equity of resource distribution among different populations, geographical locations, and specific interventions. The SIDILAC project in Latin America has refined a method to track both public expenditures and out-of-pocket costs for HIV/AIDS within country budgets (Marais and Wilson for Joint United Nations Programmme on HIV/AIDS, 2002). Analysis of the data has demonstrated serious misallocations of resources. The Latin America region, for example, significantly underspends on prevention efforts. In eight countries in the region, less than one-third of HIV/AIDS spending is directed toward public health and prevention. Even more worrisome is the gross underspending on key vulnerable groups, such as bisexual men and women, commercial sex workers, and injection-drug users, even though these vulnerable populations ultimately accounted for a large proportion of new cases of infection (Marais and Wilson, 2002). One of the most worrisome aspects of resource tracking data, however, is the unmasking of possible corruption or the diversion of funds into other activities for which donations were not intended. All of these tensions can complicate credible analysis of resource flows within M&E programs.

Over the past five years, resources have dramatically increased for a number of specific diseases. One major example is the Global Fund, which now has more than US$5 billion pledged to fight tuberculosis, malaria, and HIV/AIDS. The recently announced U.S. President's Emergency Plan for AIDS Relief has pledged US$15 billion over the next five years (2004 to 2008), and several major European donors have also increased their development assistance for health issues. With these new initiatives, we are witnessing a shift in methods of funds disbursement. There is now an increasing requirement for performance- or results-based financial disbursements. Funding will be carefully tied to specific, time-limited achievement of indicators and targets, and the next transfer of monies will not occur unless these reports are received and predefined targets achieved. Depending on donor flexibility and contractual language, overspecifying deliverables and time frames at project initiation may preclude program adjustments that might be necessary based on early and ongoing feedback. Although many donors in the past have stated that accountability is part of the funding process, such close linking of results to funding renewal is unprecedented. Pressure that currently exists to perform and report on specified targets can be overwhelming, particularly in low-resource settings, where health care and community services are experiencing resource-capacity constraints and may be on the verge of collapse.

An example of the negative effects of such results-based disbursement systems can be seen in the recent experience of the Global Alliance for Vaccines and Immunizations. Financial incentives were linked to meeting and exceeding immunization coverage statistics (numbers or percentages of targeted people who were actually immunized within a specified time frame). External auditing of the reported service statistics demonstrated a high rate of inaccuracy, with numbers far in excess of reality. In response to this perceived problem, the Global Alliance for Vaccines and Immunizations is now combining self-reported data with selective external audits to better assess the data quality and results.

As most national health services move toward decentralization and empowerment of local health enterprises for the delivery of health services, service delivery data can produce a potentially negative environment for accurate reporting. Resource allocation and policy decisions are both influenced by central government and local authorities with emphasis on cost containment, sometimes at the expense of retaining human resources. Emphasis on cost containment in already resource-strapped environments may exacerbate an environmental tendency toward reporting inaccuracy because of workforce demoralization (Kapiriri, Norheim, and Heggenhougen, 2003).

When the health system is decentralized as part of more general reform of the system, reform of health management and services also occurs. The health system reform in Zambia is an example. In that effort, it soon became clear that central health services management and political capacity lacked transparency where planning and implementation of policies and resource allocation were concerned. When this capacity was transferred to regional levels, it became obvious that transparency and not a lack of ideas or concepts was the problem in tracking the epidemic (Stekelenburg and Peeperkorn, 2004). On the other hand, when local systems are open to scrutiny through surveys that measure service coverage and quality of work, potentially "punitive" action may result. Budget-related performance indicators such as operational plans and service deliverables that do not meet expected levels (or nonperformance) may result in policy or program shifts, human resource changes, and increased pressure to deliver (Government of Malawi, 2002). Establishing structures for inclusive, participatory planning with subnational health providers who are granted selected decision-making and priority-setting powers may contribute to eliminating threats and maintaining the accuracy of facility-based surveys.

Individual Versus Community Rights: Role of Confidentiality

The inherent tension between individual rights and public good is not an issue unique to AIDS. Historical references to cholera, typhoid, and the plague tell of the use of quarantines, expulsions, denial of human rights, restrictions from accessing legal protections, and physical abuse. Although infrequently invoked, U.S. public health officials may at their discretion and in the public's interest involuntarily quarantine patients who have tuberculosis or smallpox who are not adhering to their treatment regimens (Lacey, 2003). The recent U.S. Model State Emergency Health Powers Act, passed in over twenty states, dictates the use of "the least restrictive means necessary" to protect public health (Colmers and Fox, 2003; Lacey, 2003). Furthermore, the U.S. Department of Health and Human Services "has encouraged reform of existing state public health laws" because "quarantine laws may conflict with notions of individual liberty under modern Constitutional law" (Lacey, 2003, p. 2003).

In recent debates surrounding legal authority necessary for the response to a bioterrorism threat, some have pointed to early controversy during the first decade of the HIV/AIDS epidemic about the leeway that should be granted to public health authorities. In those early years, there was an ongoing battle between the rights of individuals to refuse HIV testing or to keep HIV-positive status confidential versus the need for the public to protect itself from an impending epidemic.

In an early literature review of ethical approaches to AIDS, Manuel and others (1990) classified then-available literature into two categories: those advocating protection of society and ethical arguments in support of privileging individual rights. Measures found in that literature aimed at society's protection against AIDS include quarantine, exposure of personal medical information, criminalization of noncompliant individuals, and mandatory testing and seropositivity disclosure. Measures to protect the individual include confidentiality, prevention of discrimination due to HIV status, and free movement. Manuel and others concluded that although a perceived conflict exists between the rights of society versus the individual, "particularly as far as the confidential nature of medical information is concerned, measures intended to protect the individual also protect society" (1990, p. 14).

Tensions persist, however, when individual rights are perceived to be privileged over that of the larger society (Colmers and Fox, 2003; Schneider and Fassin, 2002). In ethical terms, HIV-testing arguments often represent conflicts between respect for persons and autonomy versus the principle of community beneficence (Macklin, 2003). For example, compelling all pregnant women to be tested for HIV is a dilemma. On the one hand, determining seropositivity can offer the fetus protection against HIV infection; on the other, it values protecting the fetus over the choices and freedoms of the woman to be tested and treated or not. van Niekerk (2001) described such complexities inherent in dealing with the epidemic, noting that they "may not be successfully addressed even through an analytical approach wherein we distinguish parts and whole, often with the expectation that addressing the parts will fix the whole" (p. 145). M&E programs, thus, must strike a balance between generating meaningful tactical-level information for program managers while taking steps to ensure public data use does not worsen discrimination and stigma experienced by those who are HIV seropositive.

Provision of HIV counseling and testing is seen as both a prevention intervention and a method of identifying cases for the purposes of initiating treatment. M&E information obtained from HIV-seroprevalence testing sites can provide valuable insights into infection prevalence among self-identified vulnerable groups. Such data may also be used to identify transmission trends within these populations. Voluntary versus mandatory testing outside of just the antenatal period has become an extremely controversial topic as access to antiretroviral therapy is scaled up in developing countries.

A major challenge to rapid treatment deployment is a targeted population's willingness to accept HIV testing. Even in countries with free access to antiretroviral therapy, much of the adult population is not ready to be tested. Reasons widely cited in the literature include stigma and discrimination, which continue to play a major role where testing is offered without adequate patient confidentiality protections against seropositivity status disclosure (Barden-O'Fallon and others, 2004; Poindexter, 2004; Savasta, 2004; Stansbury and Sierra, 2004; Kalichman and Simbayi, 2003; Parker and Aggleton, 2003; Worthington and Myers, 2003; Herek, Capitanio, and Widaman, 2002; Fullilove and Fullilove, 1999; Herek and Glunt, 1988). Partially as a result of patients' fears of involuntary serostatus disclosure, in Malawi less than 3 percent of the adult population know their HIV serostatus, making access to prevention, treatment, care and support, and future planning difficult and leaving certain program services underused (Government of Malawi, 2003). van Niekerk notes that "reinforcement of old prejudices has now shifted from individuals and communities to a whole continent. . . . AIDS is increasingly called 'the African epidemic'" (2001, p. 150).

In the protection of human rights, guidelines for HIV testing have historically maintained it must be voluntary and combined with adequate communication before testing and before results and counseling after results delivery (Manuel and others, 1990). In virtually all settings, the focus has been on enabling the individual to retain the right to refuse testing or to opt in when it is offered. Such a testing framework preserves basic individual human rights. Some have argued, however, that this preservation unnecessarily places the larger society at risk. Opponents of opt-in testing argue that if individuals are allowed to keep their seropositivity status secret, those they engage in sex with may not undertake fully informed self-protective behavioral decisions regarding transmission.

Precedent exists for HIV testing in antenatal care (ANC) settings. Often-compulsory, routine, and cost-effective antenatal urine and serum testing for syphilis, blood grouping, and hemoglobin has become the standard of care in many developed societies to protect the fetus. Furthermore, epidemiologists have used HIV prevalence in the ANC setting and among military recruits to estimate HIV seropositivity in the general population. In developed countries, the recent use of strategies for the prevention of mother-to-child transmission (MTCT)—counseling, ANC testing, short-course antiretroviral therapy, elective cesarean delivery—have yielded MTCT rates as low as 2 percent of births among HIV-infected women (Preble and Piwoz, 2001). In contrast, 25 to 35 percent of African HIV-positive women, with diminished access to such interventions, deliver an HIV-positive child (Preble and Piwoz, 2001).

Although early MTCT programs rapidly "illustrated the effective use of ANC as an entry point to care, they had also generated a cohort of HIV-infected mothers without access to treatment" (Rabkin and El-Sadr, 2003, p. 1). Based on this strategic information, MTCT programs evolved from prevention-oriented programs to prevention- and treatment-linked programs called "MTCT plus." MTCT-plus initiatives seek "to further reduce vertical transmission of HIV, and to strengthen families and communities as well as individuals" by providing antiretroviral treatment to HIV-positive women shortly before delivery and to the family thereafter (Rabkin and El-Sadr, 2003). In an era where the transmission of HIV to an unborn child can be so effectively minimized by antiretroviral treatment and other interventions, the argument surrounding routine HIV testing in pregnant women to protect an unborn child's life is probably clearer than in other nonobstetrical cases for HIV testing. Botswana, for example, has recently debated holding any doctor who does not test a pregnant woman for HIV professionally negligent (Botswana Lawyers Task Force on HIV/AIDS, 2003).

Basic human rights—the right to autonomy and the right to privacy—are not negotiable. They are enshrined in almost every constitution and protected by international conventions and agreements (United Nations General Assembly, 1948, 1966, 1979, 1989). Within these parameters, medical consent and confidentiality, as well as the right to seek, receive, and impart information on testing, may need to be adapted and redefined to suit the aims of increasing treatment access. It should always be kept in mind that the unauthorized disclosure of an individual's serological status may lead to stigma and discrimination; social isolation; estrangement of family and friends; and loss of employment, housing, and insurance.

Several questions remain in this complex and dynamic issue, such as the limits of consent and the principles of confidentiality in testing and disclosure. Ethicists, physicians, and human rights lawyers, among others, have acknowledged that exceptions may be made (Jürgens, 2001). However, the definition and extent of these concerns are a matter of grave dispute, such as the following:

- How can the line between the need for patient confidentiality and the protection of public health be better defined?
- Should there be a requirement to maintain patient confidentiality if an unsuspecting partner is at significant risk of infection?
- Is absolute confidentiality realistic?
- Should the line be extended to include the groups in society that assert a right to know the serological status of HIV-infected individuals?

Selective Use of Evaluation Data to Support Political Bias

Over the past several decades, there have been numerous examples of how the selective use of evaluation data can distort the understanding about severity of disease and the need and efficacy for specific interventions. Political consideration can be more important than epidemiological data in public health decision making (Moss, 2000). We have only to look back at the suppression of information demonstrating the serious health threat represented by tobacco and the long delays in releasing and then acting on this information when it finally became available (Muggli and Hurt, 2003).

Specific to the HIV/AIDS global crisis, data may be inaccurate, attributed to the wrong population, or threatening to political leaders. Whiteside, Barnett, George, and van Niekirk report that HIV/AIDS data have been selectively used to hide the fact that "prevention efforts [may] not have worked and there [may be] political problems of having an epidemic of this scale" (2003, p. 60). The same authors note that the problem of politically motivated selective use may be compounded by interpretations that are "simply wrong." For example, findings from Kwaramba's study examining the socioeconomic effects of HIV/AIDS on agriculture in a discrete region in Zimbabwe were misapplied by others to the whole country (Whiteside, Barnett, George, and van Niekirk, 2003). Those engaged in M&E have a professional and ethical responsibility to clearly disclaim the limits of data sources and the analyses based on them to ensure that the scale and scope of problems are as accurately portrayed as possible. Friction exists between the sense of urgency surrounding response to the HIV/AIDS epidemic and the responsibility of researchers and M&E professionals to accept and use quality data and to view it critically (Whiteside, Barnett, George, and van Niekirk, 2003).

Especially within the field of HIV/AIDS, there continue to be major concerns about the efficacy of specific interventions and the lack and credibility of the evaluation research on which they are based. In a recent report focusing on Texas, Human Rights Watch documented that government-funded "abstinence-only" programs not only keep students from receiving basic information on HIV prevention but also provide information asserting that condoms are ineffective in preventing HIV transmission (Canadian HIV/AIDS Legal Network, 2003). Data supporting views about controversial subjects like abstinence education are often lacking and inconsistent. Until such studies are conducted, debates will persist, and efforts to apply rational and proven interventions will continue to suffer.

Nowhere have these controversies been more apparent than in the debate over the efficacy of needle-exchange programs to reduce the transmission of HIV and the hepatitis C virus. A review of the available data shows that needle-exchange programs combined with other "harm-reduction" efforts can usually, but not always, be effective in limiting HIV transmission among injection-drug users. Continuing research is clearly needed regarding how to maximize the availability of sterile injection equipment and how to integrate this with other needed health and social services. Recently, the criticisms of needle exchange have been largely based not on epidemiological data but on the symbolic meaning of needle-exchange programs. These programs are said to "condone drug use" and "send the wrong message about drug use." Similar arguments are advanced by those objecting to the distribution of condoms, lubricant, and clean injecting supplies to inmates in prisons, despite scientific evidence that the use of these measures decreases the spread of HIV (May and Williams, 2002). Illustrating the triumph of politics and ideology over science, condoms are available in less than 1 percent of U.S. jails and prisons (May and Williams, 2002). These value conflicts have greatly hampered the collection of relevant data and have shifted the grounds for opposition from scientific criteria to the symbolic meaning (Des Jarlais, 2000).

The lack of convincing empirical data can foster an environment where value judgments dominate over evidence. It should also be noted that the actual conducting of controversial research is restricted. Recently in the United States, political lobbying groups were able to successfully request the National Institutes of Health to investigate a list of U.S. researchers who were engaged in studies on birth control, sex, drug use, AIDS, and sexually transmitted infections (Editors of *Lancet,* 2004). In addition to conducting the needed research, efficient peer review processes to assess these studies are critical. In 2000, the U.S. Congress enacted the Data Quality Act and directed the White House Office of Management and Budget to develop guidelines to ensure the quality of data disseminated by the federal government. Whereas the goal of improving the assessment of the credibility of research studies and dissemination of such information may be worthy, there are, nevertheless, substantial concerns. If the peer review process is too unwieldy and burdensome, a form of gridlock may occur in which nothing gets accomplished because the scientific basis of any potentially controversial piece of information or regulation is continually being challenged (Steinbrook, 2004; Whiteside, Barnett, George, and van Niekirk, 2003).

Conclusions

Although it is easy to criticize the negative influences on accurate monitoring that are presented in this chapter, it must always be remembered that public health issues and our monitoring of them occur in a real world. Protecting the reputation and economic status of one's country is not a minor issue. With the continued lack of critical evaluation research on the efficacy of various interventions, it is understandable that politicians and program planners will seize on the limited available data that best support their personal views. The concerns that have been presented in this chapter can be addressed in a number of ways.

To address the effects of stigma and denial and the tensions over data use, the positive influence of major international consensus-building forums and the drafting of universal commitments signed by member nations should not be underestimated. Chapter Three in this issue presents the groundbreaking effort of drafting the UNGASS Declaration of Commitment; establishing a set of "core indicators"; adopting routine reporting requirements; and the subsequent effects on increasing commitment for routine, standardized M&E across countries. Increased involvement of stakeholders at all levels, especially civil society, can improve the accuracy and use of such data. Serving as monitors of the quality and availability of specific data, community members and nongovernmental organizations can play a powerful role in furthering the gathering and disseminating of essential information about the epidemic and the services that are currently provided.

Furthermore, as the need for clinical service delivery and coverage data increases, it will be important that staff who deliver important services are part of the process of developing these monitoring systems and that assurances are provided that they will not be penalized for reporting accurately on numbers served. This culture of using data to improve and not to punish will take time to establish.

The issue of attributing results directly to the resources from a specific donor is complex and requires careful consideration. It is understandable that a major donor and leader in the global response to the HIV/AIDS pandemic be able to demonstrate the effects of its funds. However, as we measure outcome and impact indicators, such as coverage of antiretroviral therapy and assessment of improved survival and quality of life for persons receiving treatment, there are political, strategic, and logistical reasons to address attribution carefully. Rarely are these outcomes attributable to a single donor. It should be possible to describe their leadership role and the effects of major funding provided under the donor community and to also foster a culture of collective responsibility for actions and the desire to measure collective achievements.

Increased funding for program implementation can play an important role in enhancing the focus on accountability and the systems to measure performance. The Global Fund and other new initiatives provide a unique opportunity to advance the implementation and quality of M&E and facilitate the appropriate and transparent use of data. Not only are performance-based disbursement mechanisms a driving force to provide improved collection of data to ensure the next round of funding, but these new sources of revenue can also be used to support M&E activities. Now for the first time since the beginning of the epidemic, we may have the political commitment, the technical tools, and the financial resources to adequately support M&E.

It is essential to prove that timely, accurate, and relevant data can be seen to serve rather than to harm programs. As M&E programs are established or strengthened at the national and subnational levels, political bodies must be brought into the dialogue. HIV is politically charged in most countries. Important religious and political lobbies, along with the general population, may oppose specific interventions. It is in this context that M&E is perhaps most useful of all. Only careful measuring and recording of the success of existing initiatives will persuade reluctant policymakers to expand program efforts further (Joint United Nations Programmme on HIV/AIDS, 2000).

References

Abbasi, K. "BSE Inquiry Plays Down Errors." *British Medical Journal,* 2000, *321,* 1097.

Arndt, C., and Lewis, J. D. "The Macroeconomic Implications of HIV/AIDS in South Africa: A Preliminary Assessment." World Bank. Paper presented to the International AIDS Economics Network Conference, Durban, South Africa, July 2000.

Barden-O'Fallon, J. L., and others. "Factors Associated with HIV/AIDS Knowledge and Risk Perception in Rural Malawi." *AIDS and Behavior,* 2004, *2*(8), 131–140.

Blackburn, E. "Bioethics and the Political Distortion of Biomedical Science." *New England Journal of Medicine,* 2004, *350*(14), 1379–1380.

Botswana Lawyers Task Force on HIV/AIDS. *Routine or Compulsory Testing in Botswana?* Gaberone: Botswana Lawyers Task Force on HIV/AIDS, 2003.

Burkhalter, H. "The Politics of AIDS: Engaging Conservative Activists." *Foreign Affairs,* 2004, *83*(1), 8–14.

Canadian HIV/AIDS Legal Network. " 'Abstinence Only Until Marriage': US Approach Undermining HIV Prevention." *Canadian HIV/AIDS Policy and Law Review,* 2003, *8*(1), 37.

Choi, K. H., Gibson, D. R., Han, L., and Guo, Y. "High Levels of Unprotected Sex with Men and Women Among Men Who Have Sex with Men: A Potential Bridge of HIV Transmission in Beijing, China." *AIDS Education and Prevention,* 2004, *16*(1), 19–30.

Cohen, D. *Human Capital and the HIV Epidemic in Sub-Saharan Africa.* Geneva: International Labour Orgnization Program on HIV/AIDS and the World of Work, 2002.

Colmers, J. M., and Fox, D. M. "The Politics of Emergency Health Powers and the Isolation of Public Health." *American Journal of Public Health,* 2003, *93*(3), 397–399.

Debt, AIDS, Trade, Africa (DATA). "G8 and African Leadership in the War on AIDS and Extreme Poverty." 2004. [http://www.data.org/archives/G82004report.pdf]. Accessed June 17, 2004.

Des Jarlais, D. "Research, Politics, and Needle Exchange." *American Journal of Public Health,* 2000, *90*(9), 1392–1394.

Drazen, J. M. "SARS–Looking Back over the First 100 Days." *New England Journal of Medicine,* 2003, *349*(4), 319–320.

Durban Declaration. "HIV Causes AIDS: Curbing the Spread of This Virus Must Remain the First Step Towards Eliminating This Devastating Disease." *Nature,* 2000, 406, 15–16. (Electronic version).

Epstein, S. *Impure Science: AIDS, Activism and the Politics of Knowledge.* Berkeley: University of California Press, 1996. [http://texts.cdlib.org/dynaxml/servlet/d ynaXML?docId=ft1s20045x&chunk.id=d0e1152]. Accessed June 17, 2004.

Fox, D. M. "Comment: Epidemiology and the New Political Economy of Medicine." *American Journal of Public Health,* 1999, *89*(4), 493–496.

Fullilove, M., and Fullilove, R. "Stigma as an Obstacle to AIDS Action." *American Behavioral Scientist,* 1999, *42,* 1117–1129.

Government of Malawi. *The Impact of HIV/AIDS on Human Resources in the Malawi Public Sector.* Lilongwe: Government of Malawi, 2002.

Government of Malawi. "National HIV/AIDS Policy: A Call for Renewed Action." Office of the President and Cabinet, National AIDS Commission, 2003. [http://www.sarpn. org.za/documents/d0000702/index.php]. Accessed June 17, 2004.

Gow, J. "The HIV/AIDS Epidemic in Africa: Implications for U.S. Policy." *Health Affairs,* 2002, *21*(3), 57–69.

Herek, G. M., Capitanio, J. P., and Widaman, K. F. "HIV-Related Stigma and Knowledge in the United States: Prevalence and Trends, 1991–1999." *American Journal of Public Health,* 2002, *92,* 371–377.

Herek, G. M., and Glunt, E. K. "An Epidemic of Stigma: Public Reactions to AIDS." *American Psychiatry,* 1988, *43,* 886–891.

Human Rights Watch. *Just Die Quietly: Domestic Violence and Women's Vulnerability to HIV in Uganda.* New York: Human Rights Watch, 2003.

Human Rights Watch. *Nigeria's 2003 Elections: The Unacknowledged Violence.* New York: Human Rights Watch, 2004a.

Human Rights Watch. *Turning a Blind Eye: Hazardous Child Labor in El Salvador's Sugarcane Cultivation.* New York: Human Rights Watch, 2004b.

Jamison, T., Sachs, J., and Wang, J. "The Effect of the AIDS Epidemic on Economic Welfare in Sub-Saharan Africa." Commission on Macroeconomics and Health, Working Paper Series Paper No. WG1: 13, 2001.

Joint United Nations Programme on HIV/AIDS and others. "National AIDS Programs—A Guide to Monitoring and Evaluation." UNAIDS/00.17E. June 2000. [http:// www.unisa.org].

Jürgens, R. *HIV Testing and Confidentiality: Final Report.* (2nd ed.) Montréal: Canadian HIV/AIDS Legal Network and Canadian AIDS Society, 2001.

Kalichman, S. C., and Simbayi, L. C. "HIV Testing Attitudes, AIDS Stigma, and Voluntary HIV Counselling and Testing in a Black Township in Cape Town, South Africa." *Sexually Transmitted Infections,* 2003, *79,* 442–447.

Kapiriri, L., Norheim, O. F., and Heggenhougen, K. "Public Participation in Health Planning and Priority Setting at the District Level in Uganda." *Health Policy and Planning,* 2003, *18*(2), 205–213.

Lacey, C. "Abuse of Quarantine Authority: The Case for a Federal Approach to Infectious Disease Containment." *Journal of Legal Medicine,* 2003, *24,* 199–214.

Lacey, R. W. *Mad Cow Disease: The History of BSE in Britain.* St. Helier, Jersey, U.K.: Gypsela, 1994.

"Keeping Ideology and Bureaucracy Out of Science [editorial]." *Lancet,* 2004, *323*(9408), 501.

Laswell, H. D. *Politics: Who Gets What, When and How.* New York: Meridian, 1958.

Macklin, R. "Applying the Four Principles." *Journal of Medical Ethics,* 2003, *29,* 275–280.

Manuel, C., and others. "The Ethical Approach to AIDS: A Bibliographical Review." *Journal of Medical Ethics,* 1990, *16*(1), 14–27.

Marais, H., and Wilson, A., for Joint United Nations Programme on HIV/AIDS. "Meeting the Need." In Report on the Global HIV/AIDS Epidemic. Geneva: Joint United Nations Programme on HIV/AIDS, 2002.

May, J. P., and Williams, E. L., Jr. "Acceptability of Condom Availability in a U.S. Jail." AIDS Education and Prevention, 2002, 14(5 suppl. B), 85–91.

Moss, A. R. "Epidemiology and the Politics of Needle Exchange." American Journal of Public Health, 2000, 90, 1385–1387.

Muggli, M. E., and Hurt, R. D. "Tobacco Industry Strategies to Undermine the Eighth World Conference on Tobacco or Health." Tobacco Control, 2003, 12, 195–202.

Parker, R. "The Global HIV/AIDS Pandemic, Structural Inequalities, and the Politics of International Health." American Journal of Public Health, 2002, 92(3), 1385–1387.

Parker, R., and Aggleton, P. "HIV and AIDS-Related Stigma and Discrimination: A Conceptual Framework and Implications for Action." Social Science and Medicine, 2003, 57, 13–24.

Parry, J. "WHO Warns That Avian Flu Could Still Be in the Environment in Hong Kong." British Medical Journal, 2004, 328, 426.

Peterson, A. "Fighting AIDS in Uganda: What Went Right?" Hearing before the Subcommittee on African Affairs of the Committee on Foreign Relations, U.S. Senate, 108th Congress, Panel 1, 2003. [http://foreign.senate.gov/testimony/2003/Petersontestimony030519.pdf]. Accessed June 17, 2004.

Poindexter, C. C. "Medical Profiling: Narratives of Privilege, Prejudice, and HIV Stigma." Qualitative Health Research, 2004, 14(4), 496–512.

Preble, E. A., and Piwoz, E. G. "Prevention of Mother-to-Child Transmission of HIV in Africa: Practical Guidance for Programs." From Support for Analysis and Research in Africa (SARA) Project. 2001. [http://www.aed.org/publications/healthpublications/mtctjuly17.pdf]. Accessed June 17, 2004.

Rabkin, M., and El-Sadr, W. M. "Saving Mothers, Saving Families: The MTCT-Plus Initiative." In MTCT-Plus Initiative at the Mailman School of Public Health, Columbia University, MTCT Plus Summary (WHO Case Study). 2003. [http://www.mtctplus.org/resources.html]. Accessed June 17, 2004.

Reilly, B., Van Herp, M., Sermand, D., and Dentico, N., for Médécins sans Frontières. "SARS and Carlo Urbani." New England Journal of Medicine, 2003, 348(20), 1951–1952.

Sabatier, R. Blaming Others: Prejudice, Race and Worldwide AIDS. London: Panos, 1988.

Savasta, A. M. "HIV: Associated Transmission Risks in Older Adults: An Integrative Review of the Literature." Journal of the Association of Nurses in AIDS Care, 2004, 15(1), 50–59.

Schneider, H., and Fassin, D. "Denial and Defiance: A Socio-Political Analysis of AIDS in South Africa." AIDS, 2002, 16(suppl. 4), S45-S51.

Scott, S., and Duncan, C. J. Biology of Plagues: Evidence From Historical Populations. Cambridge: Cambridge University Press, 2001.

Stansbury, J. P., and Sierra, M. "Risks, Stigma and Honduran Garifuna Conceptions of HIV/AIDS." Social Science and Medicine, 2004, 59, 457–471.

Steinbrook, R. "Peer Review and Federal Regulations." New England Journal of Medicine, 2004, 350, 2.

Stekelenburg, R., and Peeperkorn, R. (coproducers and codirectors). "Health Reforms at Work: Experiences with Sector-Wide Approach in Zambia" [motion picture]. Amsterdame: Netherlands, 2004 (Available from the authors).

Transparency International. Global Corruption Report 2004. London: Transparency International, 2004.

United Nations Children's Fund. Africa's Orphaned Generations. New York: United Nations Children's Fund, 2003a.

United Nations Children's Fund. A League Table of Child Maltreatment Deaths in Rich Nations. New York: United Nations Children's Fund, 2003b.

United Nations Development Fund. *Gender Focused Responses to HIV/AIDS in Swaziland.* New York: United Nations Development Fund, 2002.

United Nations General Assembly. Article 19 in United Nations General Assembly Resolution 217 A (III). *Universal Declaration of Human Rights.* 1948. [http://www.un.org/Overview/rights.html]. Accessed June 17, 2004.

United Nations General Assembly. Article 19.2 in United Nations General Assembly Resolution 2200A (XXI.) *International Covenant on Civil and Political Rights.* 1966. [http://www.unhchr.ch/html/menu3/b/a_ccpr.htm]. Accessed June 17, 2004.

United Nations General Assembly. Article 10 in United Nations General Assembly Resolution 34/180. *Convention on the Elimination of All Forms of Discrimination Against Women (CEDAW).* 1979. [http://www.un.org/womenwatch/daw/cedaw/econvention.htm#article10]. Accessed June 17, 2004.

United Nations General Assembly. Articles 13, 17, and 24 in United Nations General Assembly Resolution 44/25. *Convention on the Rights of the Child.* 1989. [http://www.unhchr.ch/html/menu3/b/k2crc.htm]. Accessed June 17, 2004.

U.S. Agency for International Development. *Children on the Brink-A Joint Report on Orphan Estimates and Program Strategies.* Washington, D.C.: USAID, UNICEF, and UNAIDS, 2002

U.S. Central Intelligence Agency. "Uganda." In *The World Factbook 2004.* [http://www.cia.gov/cia/publications/factbook/geos/ug.html]. Accessed June 17, 2004.

van Niekerk, A. A. "Moral and Social Complexities of AIDS in Africa." *Journal of Medicine and Philosophy,* 2001, 27(2), 143–162.

Wald, K. D., Button, J. W., and Rienzo, B. A. "Morality Politics vs. Political Economy: The Case for School-Based Health Centers." *Social Science* Quarterly, 2001, 82(2), 221–234.

Watts, J. "China Faces Up to HIV/AIDS Epidemic: World AIDS Day Is Marked by Launch of Huge Public-Awareness Campaign." *Lancet,* 2003, 362(9400), 1983.

Whiteside, A., Barnett, T., George, G., and van Niekirk, A. A. "Through a Glass Darkly: Data and Uncertainty in the Debate." *Developing World Bioethics,* 2003, 3(1), 49–76.

Worthington, C., and Myers, T. "Factors Underlying Anxiety in HIV Testing: Risk Perceptions, Stigma and Patient-Provider Power Dynamic." *Qualitative Health Research,* 2003, 13(5), 636–655.

Ziegler, P. *The Black Death.* Stroud, Gloucestershire, U.K.: Alan Sutton, 1991. (Originally published 1969.)

Zuger, A. "What Did We Learn from AIDS?" *New York Times,* Nov. 11, 2003, p. F8.

PAUL DE LAY *is the director of monitoring and evaluation for the Joint United Nations Programme on HIV/AIDS, based in Geneva, Switzerland.*

VALERIE MANDA *is a research officer for the Joint United Nations Programme on HIV/AIDS, based in Geneva, Switzerland.*

2

National programs for AIDS need the capacity to conduct their own monitoring and evaluation, not only for monitoring the epidemic and reporting to donors, but also for improving the programs.

Global Advances in Monitoring and Evaluation of HIV/AIDS: From AIDS Case Reporting to Program Improvement

Deborah Rugg, Michel Carael, Jan Ties Boerma, John Novak

The cornerstone of a country's response to the human immunodeficiency virus-acquired immunodeficiency syndrome (HIV/AIDS) epidemic is the development of an appropriate and efficient monitoring and evaluation (M&E) system. Such a system is essential to make optimal use of limited resources and integrate lessons learned with the response required for scaling up HIV/AIDS programs to achieve national-level effects (Chan Kam, Goodridge, and Moodie, 2001). If there is to be a sustainable, effective national response, national governments must be responsible for setting the agenda, leading the strategic planning process, and coordinating action. An M&E plan needs to be intricately linked to the planning and implementation of programs and ideally needs to be put in place from the start (Rugg and Mills, 2001). These concepts and approaches are not new and certainly not unique to the field of HIV/AIDS. What is unique to HIV/AIDS, however, are the following characteristics:

- AIDS is a relatively new viral disease that emerged in the early 1980s and rapidly spread within high-risk populations and subsequently within the general population in many countries
- Changes in the HIV/AIDS programming are rapid and often dramatic as progress continues to be made in understanding the origin and dynamics of HIV; the causes and patterns of HIV infection; and how we can prevent, treat, and potentially cure the disease

NEW DIRECTIONS FOR EVALUATION, no. 103, Fall 2004 © Wiley Periodicals, Inc.

As De Lay, Ernberg, and Stanecki (2001) have stressed:

HIV/AIDS is now the fourth leading cause of death worldwide, and the single leading cause of death in sub-Saharan Africa. We have continued to be surprised, shocked and devastated by this pandemic, which the global community has consistently underestimated [p. vii].

The rapid spread of HIV has resulted in global, national, and local responses that have evolved considerably over time. Piot, the executive director of Joint United Nations Programme on HIV/AIDS (UNAIDS), has commented:

In 20 years of responses to the AIDS pandemic the world has learned many hard lessons. We have learned that half-measures do not work: progress is made only when communities and nations whole-heartedly embrace the fight against AIDS. We have learned that there is no "one-size-fits-all" solution in designing and delivering the most effective prevention and care initiatives. We have learned that HIV feeds on social inequality, especially the inequality between men and women. Above all, we have learned that we are not powerless to change the course of the pandemic. Reversing the AIDS pandemic is about changing the world we live in–our behaviors and relationships, where money flows and who makes decisions. It requires every one of us to play our part [2001, p. v].

We have come to a time when the global community has pledged an unprecedented commitment to fighting HIV/AIDS and made a concerted effort to strengthen the associated M&E systems, as illustrated by the chapters in this issue. In this chapter, we take a broad and historical look at international developments over the past twenty years in HIV/AIDS M&E. Although not intended to be exhaustive, the chapter presents epidemiological surveillance and program M&E as distinct but complementary components of a comprehensive M&E system.

One of the major shortcomings in the HIV/AIDS response has been the fragmentation of M&E efforts across various agencies. Recently, however, agencies have taken deliberate steps toward creating a unified approach that links different data collection efforts and information systems. Another major challenge is the gap that remains between the collection of data and their actual use both to reduce people's exposure to HIV infection and to improve the lives of those infected. Ideally, data use is not an isolated activity but the final stage in an interconnected series of steps, beginning with planning health information systems and continuing through collecting, managing, and analyzing data (World Health Organization, 2004a). We examine these critical data use issues and conclude with a discussion of lessons learned and the way forward.

What Do We Need to Know?

Although much of the early data collection efforts did not involve the use of a framework, an organizing framework has since evolved. The organizing M&E framework for HIV/AIDS builds on the "Framework for Program Evaluation in Public Health" (Centers for Disease Control and Prevention, 1999) and the UNAIDS' *National AIDS Programs: A Guide to Monitoring and Evaluation* (2000).

The investigation of any problem starts by asking pertinent questions that serve to initiate and organize the response. Such questions might include: What is the problem? What is contributing to the problem? What can be done about the problem? Once a program response has been implemented, is it working? and Once a reasonable period of time has passed, is the program reaching enough people to make a difference in the resolution (or severity) of the problem? (Centers for Disease Control and Prevention, 1999; Teutsch and Churchill, 1994). These basic questions provide a simple and pragmatic way to organize the resources necessary to build a national M&E system. Figure 2.1 frames the questions that must be addressed when planning a comprehensive national M&E system and considering the data sources and methods that may be employed to provide the answers. Each step in the staircase diagram is the foundation for the next step in the investigative process. Because evaluators beyond HIV/AIDS may find it useful, we will expand on this.

The first step is problem identification. In the case of HIV/AIDS, we initially seek to *identify the nature, magnitude, and course of the overall epidemic* and related subepidemics. This information typically comes from surveillance systems, special surveys, and epidemiological studies. This first step may also include questions about the *nature and magnitude of the programmatic response* to date. Situation analysis, gap analysis, and response analysis are the typical information-gathering activities that seek information about program status from, for example, related documents, informant interviews, and field observations. The methods used in this first step are also used in the last step when we determine overall impact and collective effectiveness of combined program efforts at the national level, thus closing the loop in the iterative process of program planning, implementation, and evaluation.

In the second step, we seek to determine the *contributing factors* and determinants of risk for infection. This information is usually obtained from knowledge, attitude, and behavior surveys; epidemiological risk factor studies; and determinants research. The results at this step help in the design of appropriate interventions.

The third step focuses on *what interventions might work* under ideal circumstances in rigorous research-driven protocols (efficacy trials) or under specific field conditions (effectiveness studies). This is an important

Figure 2.1. A Public Health Questions Approach to Unifying HIV/AIDS Monitoring and Evaluation

Determining Collective Effectiveness	Outcomes and Impacts Monitoring	Are collective efforts being implemented on a large enough scale to impact the epidemic (coverage; impact)? Surveys and Surveillance
Monitoring and Evaluating National Programs	Outcomes	Are interventions working/making a difference? Outcome Evaluation Studies
	Outputs	Are we implementing the program as planned? Outputs Monitoring
	Activities	What are we doing? Are we doing it right? Process Monitoring and Evaluation, Quality Assessments
Understanding Potential Responses	Inputs	What interventions and resources are needed? Needs, Resource, Response Analysis and Input Monitoring
		What interventions can work (efficacy and effectiveness)? Are we doing the right things? Special studies, Operations res., Formative res. and Research synthesis
		What are the contributing factors? Determinants Research
Problem Identification		What is the problem? Situation Analysis and Surveillance

step, although it is often not sufficiently funded in the rush to "do something" (see Chapter Nine, this issue). Typical evaluation methods include intervention outcome studies with control or comparison groups, operations research, health services research, formative research, and other special studies.

The fourth step involves determining *what specific interventions and resources are needed.* This question is usually addressed through analysis of program coverage data from special surveys or from the national health management information system. However, both sources are not fully employed at this time and will need considerable strengthening to be useful in strategic planning and management of programs. Several donors have committed to devoting extra resources in this area.

The fifth step seeks to *assess the quality of program implementation* by asking questions regarding it. Process monitoring, evaluations, and other forms of quality assessments are typically performed at this step.

Similarly, the sixth step seeks to *examine the extent of program outputs,* answering questions of "how many" and whether the program is implemented as planned. Typically this information is routinely collected from health management information systems.

The seventh step examines program outcomes and answers questions about program effectiveness. Typically, applied outcome evaluations studies are employed at this stage.

The final step focuses on determining overall program effects and collective effectiveness. Building on the answers to the questions at previous steps, information from population-based surveys and other surveillance

Figure 2.2. Global HIV/AIDS Monitoring and Evaluation Framework

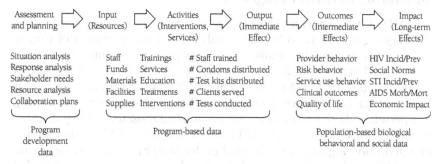

In addition to monitoring these illustrative data types, select programs conduct enhanced process and outcome evaluations.

Note: Abbreviations: STI, sexually transmitted infection; Incid/Prev, incidence or prevalence; Morb/Mort, morbidity or mortality.

activities are once again used to answer questions at this final step. In addition, the systematic collection of program-related qualitative data assists in interpreting program outcomes and impact and contributes to our understanding of what is or is not working. Such information could also identify unexpected results and community perceptions that influence program results but cannot be answered using trend data alone. However, qualitative studies are not routinely funded. This is an ongoing problem—not unique either to developing countries or to HIV/AIDS, although several donors are now planning to support such efforts.

Central Organizing Framework and Data Needed

All agencies endorse a simple "input-activities-output-outcome-impact" framework as the basic organizing framework. This provides a way to organize the data required to monitor program progress and suggests a logical order for collecting and analyzing information. The process starts with examining the required inputs (for example, resources) for implementing activities, the activities themselves (for example, counseling and testing), and then the resulting outputs (immediate effects, such as number of people tested). Outputs may lead to outcomes (intermediate effects, such as risk behavior change) that in turn may lead to impact (long-term effects, such as reduction in HIV incidence). Figure 2.2 shows this paradigm with some illustrative types of data that might be collected at each step. To truly determine the merit or value of a program, evaluation studies must supplement monitoring data, as discussed earlier.

Monitoring HIV/AIDS Programs

AIDS Case Reporting. Disease monitoring or surveillance is defined as the ongoing systematic collection, analysis, and interpretation of data to describe diseases and their transmission in populations (Centers for Disease Control and Prevention, 2003). Historically, HIV/AIDS surveillance began in the United States in 1981 with the first AIDS case definition: "a disease, at least moderately predictive of a defect in cell-mediated immunity, occurring in a person with no known cause for diminished resistance to that disease" (Centers for Disease Control and Prevention, 1982, p. 507). Although this first definition highlights the limited understanding of the disease at that time, AIDS case reporting allowed the elucidation of risk groups, provided information on sex and age patterns of the disease, suggested the various routes of transmission, and gave a general idea of where to target prevention efforts (Centers for Disease Control and Prevention and others, 2004).

In 1985, the World Health Organization (WHO) published a case definition for AIDS in Africa, the Bangui, Central African Republic, definition, which included the presence of two major signs *and* one minor associated symptom (World Health Organization, 1985). This definition was widely adopted but lacked sensitivity. However, the major limitation was that of severe underreporting (an estimated 90 percent or more of AIDS cases were not reported). Also, it was often confused with clinical staging of the disease and did not adequately capture HIV-related morbidity. Given these challenges, the AIDS case definition has subsequently been updated several times to incorporate new developments in HIV diagnostics and an increased understanding of the spectrum of morbidity associated with HIV infection.

HIV Sentinel Surveillance. When the HIV antibody test became available in 1985, it dramatically decreased reliance on AIDS case reporting for surveillance purposes. As the capacity for HIV testing became more widespread, HIV sentinel surveillance became the cornerstone of national surveillance systems. National governments and international agencies increasingly relied on HIV sentinel surveillance to provide an estimate of HIV prevalence in the general population.

The early global response to HIV/AIDS was coordinated by the WHO's Global Program on HIV/AIDS, and between 1987 and 1991, more than 145 national AIDS programs were established in resource-constrained countries around the world. Because virtually all national AIDS programs resided within ministries of health, the first national short- and medium-term plans were focused exclusively on the health sector response to the epidemic. In conjunction with advances in HIV testing capability, the WHO's Global Program on HIV/AIDS in 1987 developed guidelines for HIV surveillance among pregnant women attending antenatal clinics. The HIV prevalence among these women is still used to estimate the prevalence of HIV infection among 15- to 49-year-olds in countries with generalized epidemics (that is, HIV prevalence exceeds 1 percent in antenatal clinic clients). Many countries developed antenatal clinic-based surveillance systems, and some countries expanded these to include surveillance among other easily accessible groups, such as patients in sexually transmitted disease clinics, blood donors, and clients of voluntary counseling and testing centers. Some of these groups, however, may be biased toward higher prevalence rates largely because of higher levels of risky sexual behavior (World Health Organization, 2004b).

Behavioral Surveys. In 1988, the WHO Global Program on AIDS launched a program of surveys to collect basic descriptive information about individual perceptions, knowledge, attitudes, and sexual behaviors in general populations as they relate to the risk of HIV infection (World Health Organization, 1988). Until then, no large representative surveys on sexual behavior had ever been undertaken in developing countries because most attention was focused on populations at high risk for contracting or transmitting HIV infection. The driving force for these surveys was the assumption that greater knowledge of sexual behavior in representative samples of the general population in different sociocultural contexts should have important implications for designing and evaluating interventions to foster necessary behavioral change to control the spread of HIV infection (Carael and others, 1995).

The challenges in conducting such surveys were enormous: collecting information on sexual behavior, especially outside stable relationships, is controversial, and the definition of the basic concepts of sexual behavior and the assessment of their validity and reliability are difficult (Carballo, Cleland, Carael, and Albrecht, 1989). The focus on sexual relations with a nonregular partner is obvious. Of all the risk factors for sexually transmitted infections (STIs), including HIV, the number of recent or lifetime (or both) sexual partners has consistently proved to be one of the most important, at least where unprotected sex is widely practiced (Andersen and others, 1991). However, the actual risk of infection depends on the overall prevalence of HIV and other STIs in particular communities and networks (Carael and others, 1995).

Although the idea of conducting sexual behavior surveys among representative samples of the general population was initially greeted with reluctance both by government officials and the research community, more than twenty countries participated in the WHO Global Program on AIDS cross-cultural survey research. Unfortunately, the information collected was only partly used for planning prevention programs and for evaluating behavioral change (Carael and others, 1995). None of the countries involved in the research program repeated the surveys or transformed them into a routine behavioral monitoring tool. Despite these difficulties, the population-based HIV/AIDS surveys proved that it is indeed possible to collect highly personal and sensitive information from individuals. However, the need remains for information from a range of data sources—including quantitative and qualitative inquiries into individual behaviors and sexual network and mixing patterns—to be interpreted together.

Second-Generation HIV Surveillance. Changes in HIV prevalence may be indicative of the long-term effect of multiple HIV/AIDS prevention programs, but it is difficult to prove that observed changes are directly linked to specific programs because other factors such as mortality, migration, and saturation of the population at risk may also contribute to changes (Asamoah-Odei, Carael, Rehle, and Schwartlander, 2001). The concept of second-generation surveillance was introduced to better measure population diversity, including populations and subpopulations at risk and their epidemiological and behavioral trends over time, especially in mature epidemics. The underlying concept of second-generation surveillance is that different epidemics need different surveillance systems. Its main elements include considering biological surveillance (HIV, AIDS, other STIs) and behavioral surveillance as integral components, depending on the stage and type of the epidemic, and it provides useful information to monitor the HIV epidemic and measure the progress of the national HIV/AIDS program (Rehle, Lazzari, Dallabetta, and Asamoah-Odei, 2004).

Two major developments in monitoring HIV-risk behaviors strengthened the capacity to follow the diversity of the epidemic. First, large-scale nationally representative demographic and health surveys, which traditionally had focused on maternal and child health and family planning, increasingly included male respondents and also added a module on HIV/AIDS. This was an important step toward standardizing indicators for monitoring behavioral changes over time. Second, behavioral sentinel surveys were developed to monitor behavioral changes in specific at-risk populations (Henry, 1996; Rehle, Lazzari, Dallabetta, and Asamoah-Odei, 2004) over time. Despite the difficulties in measuring HIV-related risk behaviors through behavioral surveys, as discussed by Carael and others (1995) and Rehle, Lazzari, Dallabetta, and Asamoah-Odei (2004), behavioral surveys have been the main source of data for identifying trends in HIV-related risk behaviors to date. However, recently the value of supplementing HIV surveillance and behavioral surveys with sound qualitative data collected through rapid ethnographic assessments has proved useful in the interpretation of HIV epidemiological data and the design of effective HIV prevention programs (Needle and others, 2003). The multimethod data-triangulation approach that this represents has long been considered valuable and has received much attention in the evaluation literature (for example, Manderson and Aaby, 1992; Trotter, 1995). Although triangulating data from multiple sources takes time and skill, it can be seen as a process of "nesting" qualitative data within a quantitative data collection plan. As such, it can greatly strengthen a public health response by enhancing the sophistication of the surveillance and monitoring efforts and by providing essential data for the design of an effective response (Needle and others, 2003).

As we get better at understanding the HIV/AIDS epidemic, it should translate into an improved ability to identify and interpret changes over time and to identify factors that in turn should lead to an improved response.

The interpretation of HIV trends will be even more challenging in the coming years as antiretroviral treatment becomes more widely available. Increased access to antiretroviral treatment will lengthen the survival time of HIV-infected people and thus may potentially alter the dynamics of HIV transmission by increasing the pool of HIV-infected people, disinhibiting prevention behaviors, and perhaps, decreasing the infectiousness of those treated through reduced viral loads (Rehle, Lazzari, Dallabetta, and Asamoah-Odei, 2004).

Evaluating HIV/AIDS Programs

Here we examine national program monitoring and program evaluation studies.

National Program Monitoring. Recognizing that the survey data were not being used effectively in guiding the national response to HIV/AIDS, the WHO in 1994 designed a more focused, country-oriented methods package for the evaluation of national AIDS programs that included a set of ten priority prevention indicators (World Health Organization, 1994; Mertens and others, 1994). Four indicators—knowledge of preventive practices, reported number of nonregular sex partners, condom use with nonregular partners, and reported STIs incidence—were part of a standard questionnaire requiring repeated surveys in the general population. Two additional indicators on STI case management and services and two on HIV and syphilis seroprevalence were to be collected through health facility surveys. The remaining indicators, condom availability at central and at peripheral system levels required record reviews and special assessments. These ten priority prevention indicators were proposed as complementary measures to HIV surveillance systems. The WHO Global Program on AIDS provided both technical support through its country program advisors and financial assistance to conduct these country-level program surveys, but fewer than twenty developing countries were interested in participating (Mehret and others, 1996; Mertens and others, 1994). However, in participating countries, the survey experience had the added benefit of mobilizing program managers, clinicians, and other professional staff to improved efforts in the areas of condom supply, case management of STIs, and interventions for behavioral change (Mertens and others, 1994).

By 1991, our understanding about the complex dynamics, determinants, and consequences of HIV infection had increased. The WHO Global Program on AIDS sought to address the epidemic through a truly multisectoral response. As useful as the early short- and medium-term plans had been for providing national AIDS programs a framework for planning and implementing a national response, the plans were viewed as "external" and inadequately addressed national needs and capacities (Chan Kam and others, 2001). In 1995, the WHO Global Program on AIDS was discontinued and replaced in 1996 by the Joint United Nations Programme on HIV/AIDS.

UNAIDS comprised several U.N. agencies, thus reflecting the shift from solely defining HIV/AIDS as a health problem to approaches addressing other social and developmental aspects.

As countries formulated national strategies to combat HIV/AIDS in a coordinated multisectoral response, program monitoring became more prominent and focused on assessing whether program activities were effectively implemented and made reasonable progress toward stated goals and objectives. Although the routine collection of such monitoring information remained overall lacking, many countries conducted medium-term reviews of their national plans, using the available program data to adjust management capacities and plan future activities. (Chapter Four on collaboration in this issue describes such a medium-term review in Cambodia.)

Recent efforts have placed program monitoring firmly on the international M&E agenda (see Chapter Six, this issue). UNAIDS has invested in the development of a data management system at the country level, the Country Response Information System (Joint United Nations Programme on HIV/AIDS, 2003) (see also Chapter Three, this issue). This system is scheduled for implementation in over one hundred countries by 2005. It can store epidemiological data, strategic planning information, budget allocation information, program description and implementation data, and a country-specific research inventory. The Country Response Information System should facilitate coordination of activities between the national government, donors, and implementing agencies to achieve adequate coverage of, and necessary synergies between, HIV/AIDS programs.

In addition, with support from the U.S. Agency for International Development, HIV/AIDS indicator data from a range of surveys conducted in a large number of countries has now been compiled in an easily accessible database (ORC Macro, 2004). Indicators from the following sources that are routinely collected through population-based surveys can be found in this database: UNAIDS *National AIDS Programs: Guide to Monitoring and Evaluation* (Joint United Nations Programme on HIV/AIDS, 2000), the indicators to monitor the United Nations General Assembly Special Session on HIV/AIDS (Joint United Nations Programme on HIV/AIDS, 2002), and the Millennium Development Goals (United Nations Development Program, 2004).

Program Evaluation Studies. As discussed earlier, several studies have used population-based cross-sectional, and longitudinal data collection methods to monitor trends both in the HIV/AIDS epidemic and, as described in Chapter Six in this issue, in the national programmatic response. These data sources have been supplemented by some studies attempting to understand behavioral change attributable to specific HIV/AIDS programs, but few of these studies have been done because of their high cost and complexity. From the perspective of a national program, as suggested by the editors previously in the discussion of the M&E pipeline (see Editors' Notes in this volume), it may not be practical, or even necessary, to assess behavioral change for every individual project, especially when those projects are using strategies with already proven effectiveness (Saidel and others, 2001). Nevertheless, there is still a need for in-depth evaluation studies that focus on the effects of new or innovative interventions. Only a few rigorous, large-scale program evaluations have been conducted to date, notably in the areas of voluntary counseling and testing, school sexual health education, and mass media communication. The voluntary counseling and testing study, for example, was a randomized trial to test the efficacy of HIV counseling and testing in reducing sexual risk behavior (Voluntary HIV-1 Counseling and Testing Efficacy Study Group, 2000). This multicountry study was conducted in 1995 to 1998 in Tanzania, Kenya, and Trinidad. Sexual behavior data collected at six- and twelve-month intervals after HIV counseling showed that the intervention was most effective for HIV-infected people and sexual partners who received the counseling as a couple. Although a cost-effective intervention, especially in urban settings, its cost-effectiveness could be significantly improved through targeted approaches, such as linking counseling and testing to other services that reach high-prevalence populations (for example, in-service sites for STIs) (Sweat and others, 2000). Other examples include the Rakai (Uganda) and Mwanza (Tanzania) studies, which investigated the relationship between the treatment of STIs and sexual transmission of HIV. A decrease in population-level HIV incidence was associated with improved case management of STIs in Mwanza but was not associated with mass treatment of STIs in Rakai (Grosskurth and others, 2000). The results of the Mwanza trial had a major influence on HIV-prevention policies in many countries around the world. How-ever, the unexpected, and seemingly contradictory, results of the Rakai trial resulted in uncertainty among policymakers and donor agencies regarding the measurable effects of interventions to reduce the incidence of STIs. Grosskurth and others (2000) argue that the results from the Mwanza and the Rakai trials are not directly comparable because they tested different interventions in different epidemiological settings using different evaluation methods. They point out that the results may be complementary, rather than contradictory, and offer possible explanations, including: differences in the stage of the HIV-1 epidemic, which can influence exposure to HIV-1 and the distribution of viral load in the infected population; potential differences in the prevalence of incurable STIs; perhaps a greater influence on HIV-1 transmission of symptomatic, rather than symptomless, STIs; and possibly greater effectiveness of continuously available services rather than intermittent mass treatment to control rapid reinfection with a sexually transmitted disease (Grosskurth and others, 2000). This example illustrates the complexities of interpreting findings from large-scale impact evaluations.

Although many more smaller-scale program evaluations have been conducted, there has been less focus on what constitutes a comprehensive evaluation agenda and on appropriate methods for evaluation (see Chapter Nine, this issue). As a result, there remain significant knowledge gaps about what programs work best for which populations.

Bringing Monitoring and Evaluation Together

In recent years, there has been an increasing effort by the international community to rapidly scale up HIV prevention, care, and treatment programs; harmonize the corresponding M&E strategies and monitoring indicators; and coordinate M&E activities so that resources are used effectively to support complementary activities. This unified approach to M&E will also reduce the burden of data collection at the country level by reducing the reporting of multiple indicators to multiple stakeholders. Over the past five years, significant advances have also been made in building the human and fiscal capacity to implement these national M&E systems. These efforts at the global level have highlighted the degree of fragmentation at the country level and, hence, the paramount need for local coordination. In a recent landmark event—spearheaded by UNAIDS, the U.S. government, the World Bank, and the Global Fund to Fight AIDS, Tuberculosis and Malaria—multiple agencies and governments met and endorsed a renewed commitment to coordination guided by a new unifying theme: the "three ones principle." This principle encourages all governments and donors working in HIV/AIDS to acknowledge and support only *one* national AIDS authority; to develop *one* overarching national strategic plan designed to organize and coordinate all donor and sector contributions; and to collaboratively develop *one* national M&E plan with dedicated personnel and resources for a single M&E organizing committee and national indicator database (Joint United Nations Programme on HIV/AIDS, 2004; also see Chapter Four, this issue).

To monitor program performance at the country level, the local national AIDS program and the various international donors typically engage in three activities: derive a limited set of program monitoring indicators, some of which overlap and some of which are specific to each agency; collaborate to endorse a unified set of national outcome and impact indicators that measure the collective effectiveness of all program partners in making progress toward national objectives; and then collect data to inform such indicators at the country level and also work collaboratively to harmonize global reporting needs with country-specific data needs. Hundreds of variables or indicators may be collected across projects at the lower levels, such as projects, districts, and so forth. Only some of these indicators need to be aggregated at the national level (for example, national AIDS program indicators [$n > 100$], UNAIDS indicators [$n = 57$]), but only UNGASS indicators ($n = 19$) are needed to monitor programs at the global level (that is, the United Nations General Assembly Special Session Declaration of the Commitment on HIV/AIDS). This is depicted in Figure 2.3 in the global indicator pyramid, which illustrates the relative relationship among the various levels of indicators.

The M&E arena has grown rapidly; yet, M&E capacity at the country level is still limited. To address this, the major donor agencies have agreed

**Figure 2.3. Global Monitoring and Evaluation Indicator Pyramid:
Levels of Indicators**

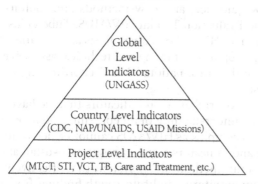

Note: UNGASS: United Nations General Assembly Special Session on HIV/AIDS; CDC: Centers for Disease Control and Prevention; NAP/UNAIDS: National AIDS Programs–Joint United Nations Programme on HIV/AIDS; USAID: U.S. Agency for International Development; MTCT: mother-to-child transmission; STI: sexually transmitted infection; TB: tuberculosis.

to jointly and systematically provide technical assistance, support the local hiring of additional M&E staff, and "learn by doing" to develop feasible approaches to building national M&E systems. For example, each agency will plan prospective evaluation studies and will also collaborate in focusing on several countries with an enhanced level of effort and technical assistance. This is a long-range collaboration (extending to at least 2008 with the current resources) with the two key goals of avoiding duplication of effort and avoiding the situation that occurred in Uganda, where answers to what actually caused the drastic reduction in HIV prevalence that occurred in the early 1990s can only be speculated upon retrospectively (Stoneburner and Low-Beer, 2004). These comprehensive longitudinal evaluation studies will provide practical information on how to implement and sustain a comprehensive yet feasible M&E system that informs national AIDS programs and donors alike on what is and is not working and where improvements are needed.

Conclusion

The past twenty years have seen an increasing awareness of the importance of M&E systems, which can provide a comprehensive understanding of the HIV/AIDS epidemic and the overall effectiveness of the resulting national response. The growing focus on collaboration epitomized in the recent "three ones principle," has fostered more progress in collaboration and more funding for M&E than ever before. This provides an unprecedented opportunity to make M&E systems work effectively in support of the national response. As treatment expands and more people receive antiretroviral therapy, there will be new issues on the agenda for effective global M&E (see Chapter Five, this issue). There will therefore be a continuous need for new standards, new indicators, new guidance, and new methods and toolkits (for example, "Monitoring and Evaluation Toolkit HIV/AIDS, Tuberculosis and Malaria," Global Fund to Fight HIV/AIDS, Tuberculosis and Malaria, 2003). This will require ongoing support for training and technical assistance to support the national AIDS authorities, national M&E coordinating committees, and program-level staff.

However, the overreliance on indicators that we have seen thus far is problematic. The understanding of an epidemic and an effective response in an epidemic as complex as HIV/AIDS cannot be determined by monitoring the disease and indicators alone. It requires a sustainable, comprehensive, strategic, multimethod M&E system that effectively integrates the information from monitoring indicators with findings from selected evaluation studies and qualitative methods that help us understand community responses to the HIV/AIDS eppidemics.

References

Andersen, R., and others. "The Spread of HIV-1 in Africa: Sexual Contact Patterns and the Predicted Demographic Impact of AIDS." *Nature,* 1991, *352,* 581–589.

Asamoah-Odei, E., Carael, M., Rehle, T., and Schwartlander, B. "Evaluation and Surveillance Approaches for HIV/AIDS Programs." In P. Lamptey and H. Gayle (eds.), *HIV/AIDS Prevention and Care in Resource-Constrained Settings: A Handbook for the Design and Management of Programs.* Arlington, Va.: Family Health International, 2001.

Carael, M., and others. "Sexual Behavior in Developing Countries: Implications for HIV Control." *AIDS,* 1995, *9,* 1171–1175.

Carballo, M., Cleland, J., Carael, M., and Albrecht, G. "A Cross National Study of Patterns of Sexual Behavior." *Journal of Sex Research,* 1989, *26*(3), 287–299.

Centers for Disease Control and Prevention. "Current Trends Update on Acquired Immune Deficiency Syndrome (AIDS)—United States." *MMWR,* Sept. 24, 1982, pp. 507–508, 513–514.

Centers for Disease Control and Prevention. "Framework for Program Evaluation in Public Health." *Morbidity and Mortality Weekly Report,* Sept. 17, 1999, pp. 1–40.

Centers for Disease Control and Prevention. *Global AIDS Program Monitoring and Evaluation Capacity Building for Program Improvement Field Guide.* Atlanta: Centers for Disease Control and Prevention, Monitoring and Evaluation Team, Global AIDS Program, 2003.

Centers for Disease Control and Prevention, U.S. Agency for International Development, WHO, UNAIDS, European Commission, and Ethiopia Public Health Association. *New Strategies for HIV/AIDS Surveillance in Resource-Constrained Countries.* Ethiopia: Addis Ababa, Jan. 26–29, 2004.

Chan Kam, C., Goodridge, G., and Moodie, R. "Strategic Planning, Program Design and Management." In P. Lamptey and H. Gayle (eds.), *HIV/AIDS Prevention and Care in Resource-Constrained Settings: A Handbook for the Design and Management of Programs.* Arlington, Va.: Family Health International, 2001.

De Lay, P., Ernberg, G., and Stanecki, K. "Introduction." In P. Lamptey and H. Gayle (eds.), *HIV/AIDS Prevention and Care in Resource-Constrained Settings: A Handbook for the Design and Management of Programs.* Arlington, Va.: Family Health International, 2001.

Global Fund to Fight HIV/AIDS, Tuberculosis and Malaria. "Monitoring and Evaluation Toolkit HIV/AIDS, Tuberculosis and Malaria (draft)." Geneva: Global Fund to Fight HIV/AIDS, Tuberculosis and Malaria, 2003.

Grosskurth, H., and others. "Control of Sexually Transmitted Diseases for HIV-1 Prevention: Understanding the Implications of the Mwanza and Rakai Trials." *Lancet,* 2000, *355*(9219), 1981–1987.

Henry, B. "BSS: Tracking Trends in Sexual Behavior." *AidsCaptions,* 1996, 3(2), 33.

Joint United Nations Programme on HIV/AIDS. *National AIDS Programs: A Guide to Monitoring and Evaluation.* Geneva: Joint United Nations Programme on HIV/AIDS, 2000.

Joint United Nations Programme on HIV/AIDS. *Country Response Information System: Overview of the System and Its Plan of Establishment.* Geneva: Joint United Nations Programme on HIV/AIDS, 2003.

Joint United Nations Programme on HIV/AIDS. "The Three Ones: Principles for the Coordination of National AIDS Responses." 2004. [http://www.unaids.org/en/about+unaids/what+is+unaids/unaids+at+country+level/the+three+ones.asp]. Accessed June 30, 2004.

Joint United Nations Programme on HIV/AIDS/United Nations General Assembly Special Session. *Guidelines on Construction of Core Indicators.* Geneva: Joint United Nations Programme on HIV/AIDS, 2002.

Manderson, L., and Aaby, P. "An Epidemic in the Field? Rapid Assessment Procedures and Health Research." *Social Science Medicine,* 1992, *35*(7), 839–850.

Mehret, M., and others. "Baseline for the Evaluation of an AIDS Program Using Prevention Indicators: A Case Study in Ethiopia." *Bulletin of the World Health Organization,* 1996, *74*, 509–516.

Mertens, T., and others. "Prevention Indicators for Evaluating the Progress of National AIDS Intervention Programs." *AIDS,* 1994, *8*, 1359–1369.

Needle, R., and others. "Rapid Assessment of the HIV/AIDS Crisis in Racial and Ethnic Minority Communities: An Approach for Timely Community Interventions." *American Journal of Public Health,* 2003, *93*, 970–979.

ORC Macro. "HIV/AIDS Indicator Survey Database." Opinion Research Corporation Co. 2004. [http://www.orcmacro.com/ProgramAreas/Health/hivaids.aspx]. Accessed June 30, 2004.

Piot, P. "Preface." In P. Lamptey and H. Gayle (eds.), *HIV/AIDS Prevention and Care in Resource-Constrained Settings: A Handbook for the Design and Management of Programs.* Arlington, Va.: Family Health International, 2001.

Rehle, T., Lazzari, S., Dallabetta, G., and Asamoah-Odei, E. "Second-Generation Surveillance: Better Data for Decision-Making." *Bulletin of the World Health Organization,* 2004, *82*(2), 1–7.

Rugg, D., and Mills, S. "Development of an Integrated Monitoring and Evaluation Plan." In T. Rehle, T. Saidel, S. Mills, and R. Magnani (eds.), *Evaluating Programs for HIV/AIDS Prevention and Care in Developing Countries.* Arlington, Va.: Family Health International, 2001.

Saidel, T., and others. "Use of Behavioral Data for Program Evaluation." In P. Lamptey and H. Gayle (eds.), *HIV/AIDS Prevention and Care in Resource-Constrained Settings: A Handbook for the Design and Management of Programs.* Arlington, Va.: Family Health International, 2001.

Stoneburner, R., and Low-Beer, D. "Population-Level HIV Declines and Behavioral Risk Avoidance in Uganda." *Science,* 2004, *304*, 714–718.

Sweat, M., and others. "Cost-Effectiveness of Voluntary HIV-1 Counseling and Testing in Reducing Sexual Transmission of HIV-1 in Kenya and Tanzania." *Lancet,* 2000, *356*, 113–121.

Teutsch, S. M., and Churchill, R. E. (eds.). *Principles and Practice of Public Health Surveillance.* New York: Oxford University Press, 1994.

Trotter, R. T. II. "Drug Use, AIDS, and Ethnography: Advanced Ethnographic Research Methods for Exploring the HIV Epidemic." NIDA Research Monographs, 1995, *157*, 38–64.

United Nations Development Program. "The Millennium Development Goals." 2004. [http://www.undp.org/ millenniumgoals]. Accessed June 30, 2004.

Voluntary HIV-1 Counseling and Testing Efficacy Study Group. "Efficacy of Voluntary HIV-1 Counseling and Testing in Individuals and Couples in Kenya, Tanzania, and Trinidad: A Randomized Trial." *Lancet*, 2000, *356*, 103–112.

World Health Organization. "Workshop on AIDS in Central Africa." World Health Organization Workshop on AIDS in Bangui, Central African Republic<\\>, 1985.

World Health Organization. *Survey on Partner Relations and Risk of HIV Infection—Phase 1*. Geneva: World Health Organization, 1988.

World Health Organization. *Evaluation of National AIDS Programs—A Methods Package*. Geneva: World Health Organization, 1994.

World Health Organization. "Guidelines for Effective Use of Data From HIV Surveillance Systems." Geneva: Joint United Nations Programme on HIV/AIDS/World Health Organization Working Group on Global HIV/AIDS/STI Surveillance, 2004a.

World Health Organization. *New Strategies for HIV/AIDS Surveillance in Resource-Constrained Countries*. Geneva: World Health Organization, 2004b.

DEBORAH RUGG *is the associate director of the Monitoring and Evaluation Team for the Global AIDS Program at the U.S. Centers for Disease Control and Prevention, Atlanta, Georgia.*

MICHEL CARAEL *retired from the chief evaluation position in the Joint United Nations Programme on HIV/AIDS in 2004 and is currently a professor at the Free University of Brussels, Belgium, and consultant in evaluation.*

JAN TIES BOERMA *is the director of the Measurement and Health Information System Section at the World Health Organization, Geneva, Switzerland.*

JOHN NOVAK *is the monitoring and evaluation adviser to the U.S. Agency for International Development, Washington D.C.*

3

The 2001 Declaration of Commitment on HIV/AIDS by 189 countries serves as a benchmark for global action. Definition of specific and time-bound targets put pressure on these countries to accelerate program implementation, but the first progress reports indicate a low response rate for some indicators and concern about data quality.

Has the United Nations General Assembly Special Session on HIV/AIDS Made a Difference?

Nicole Massoud, Paul De Lay, Michel Carael

Over the past twenty years, strategies adopted by governments affected by human immunodeficiency virus and the acquired immunodeficiency syndrome (HIV/AIDS) have gradually changed to ensure a more holistic and effective response to the epidemic. Two major shifts have occurred. Countries have moved from a strictly "health" to a "multisector" approach, and broad interventions have emerged that focus not only on the individual but also on structural issues. An increased range of actors from the civil society and the private sector have joined countries in the struggle against HIV/AIDS. In some countries, the civil society has played an instrumental role in providing a sense of urgency and conscience among stakeholders.

This sense of common purpose culminated with the adoption of a Declaration of Commitment by 189 member states, acting on behalf of governments (Joint United Nations Programme on HIV/AIDS, 2001) in June 2001 at the United Nations General Assembly Special Session on HIV/AIDS (UNGASS). The declaration covers numerous areas from leadership to resources; HIV/AIDS prevention, care, and support; and the reduction of vulnerability to exposure to HIV infection, to name a few. The declaration document still reflects the reluctance of some governments to confront sensitive issues such as high-risk behavior in certain population groups by intentionally omitting to name them and instead using vague descriptions (excerpt below). However, by addressing human rights principles, gender inequality, vulnerability, poverty, and inequity, the declaration provides a broad framework for an expanded response to the epidemic, including tailored programs for those vulnerable groups.

Definition of High-Risk Behavior Groups in the Declaration of Commitment on HIV/AIDS

Identifiable groups who currently have high or increasing rates of HIV infection or whose public health information indicates that they are at greatest risk of and most vulnerable to new infection as indicated by such factors as the local history of the epidemic, poverty, sexual practices, drug-using behavior, livelihood, institutional location, disrupted social structures and population movements, forced or otherwise.

By setting targets that are concrete and time bound and by requiring that unprecedented efforts be undertaken to measure global success in reaching these targets, the member states envisioned that the declaration would become a tool to promote greater accountability and an outcome-driven sense of urgency and solidarity in the fight against the epidemic. However, the challenge facing countries with scarce resources and weak implementation capacity is to translate the broad principles highlighted in the declaration into realistic key priorities for the short and medium terms. To assist countries in this difficult task, the Joint United Nations Programme on HIV/AIDS (UNAIDS) and its key partners developed a monitoring framework (2002a).

This chapter focuses on two topics: first, the added value of the Declaration of Commitment on HIV/AIDS and the monitoring framework for improving the national response to HIV/AIDS in member states, and second, the lessons learned from the first round of reporting with respect to the extent and quality of reporting. A discussion on the national AIDS program achievements against the declaration's targets is beyond the scope of this chapter and can be found elsewhere (Joint United Nations Programme on HIV/AIDS, 2002b, 2003a).

Unique Contribution of the Declaration of Commitment on HIV/AIDS

The UNGASS Declaration of Commitment on HIV/AIDS serves as a benchmark for global action. At international, regional, and national gatherings since the June 2001 United Nations (U.N.) special session, the declaration has helped define agendas and create a common platform for action. It has also allowed countries to review and refine their national strategic plans and to adapt the core agenda agreed upon in the declaration to the national contexts. A series of regional training workshops organized by UNAIDS and key partners assisted in the review process, placing emphasis on a single national strategy to be adopted by all players. To date, most member states have already reflected their commitment to the declaration by incorporating its agenda into their national strategic plans.

The declaration has set concrete and time-bound (that is, measurable) targets for expenditures on HIV/AIDS programs, access to education and services for youth, and reduction of HIV prevalence among youth and infants:

Measurable Targets

- By 2005, reach an overall target of annual expenditure on the epidemic of 7–10 billion United States dollars in low and middle-income countries and those countries experiencing or at risk of experiencing rapid expansion for prevention, care, treatment, support and mitigation of the impact of HIV/AIDS.
- By 2005, ensure that at least 90 percent, and by 2010 at least 95 percent, of young men and women aged 15 to 24 have access to the information, education, including peer education and youth-specific HIV education, and services necessary to develop the life skills required to reduce their vulnerability to HIV infection, in full partnership with young persons, parents, families, educators and health-care providers.
- By 2005, reduce HIV prevalence among young men and women aged 15 to 24 in the most affected countries by 25 percent and by 25 percent globally by 2010.
- By 2005, reduce the proportion of infants infected with HIV by 20 percent, and by 50 percent by 2010, by ensuring that 80 percent of pregnant women accessing antenatal care have information, counseling and other HIV-prevention services available to them.

In addition, more general targets are formulated for policies and programs on HIV/AIDS prevention, care, and support (next excerpt). Although some may appear unrealistic for a number of member states, those targets have put pressure on countries to accelerate implementation, scale up interventions, and report on progress toward their achievements.

General Targets

- By 2003, enact or strengthen policies and/or strategies on prevention, care and treatment, and human rights.
- Ensure, by 2005, that a wide range of prevention, care and support programs are available in all countries. Below, an example of general target on prevention (paragraph 52 of the Declaration):

> By 2005, ensure: that a wide range of prevention programs which take account of local circumstances, ethics and cultural values, is available in all countries, particularly the most affected countries, including information, education and communication, in languages most understood by communities and respectful of cultures, aimed at reducing

risk-taking behavior and encouraging responsible sexual behavior, including abstinence and fidelity; expanded access to essential commodities, including male and female condoms and sterile injecting equipment; harm-reduction efforts related to drug use; expanded access to voluntary and confidential counseling and testing; safe blood supplies; and early and effective treatment of sexually transmittable infections.

The declaration has also helped clarify the roles and responsibilities of all parties involved in the fight against HIV/AIDS to ensure coordinated implementation: governments, civil society, the private sector, and the United Nations system. The role of each will be discussed below. Governments are primarily responsible for implementing the declaration's agenda, including the measurement of agreed indicators and a regular review of progress toward their targets. These reviews should comprise broad-based consultation among stakeholders, their results widely disseminated, and the lessons learned used to improve programs. Donors have an additional responsibility to provide financial and technical support to the efforts of developing countries, to encourage action, and to promote the goals of the declaration in international forums.

Civil society engagement is critical to the declaration's implementation. Civil society groups act not only as powerful stimulants for national action but as influential actors in their own right. Networks of people living with HIV/AIDS or networks of people at high risk for HIV infection (such as injecting-drug users, men who have sex with men, and sex workers) are particularly important. The social mobilization necessary to achieve the declaration's goals can come only through sustained and meaningful civil society engagement.

The private sector plays an important role in the fight against HIV/AIDS and is one of the key partners in the implementation of the declaration. Ensuring its active involvement in countries where the corporate sector has remained on the sidelines so far is essential. Labor unions need to be integrated in national HIV/AIDS efforts with support from the International Labour Organization.

The U.N. system has embraced the declaration as the framework for action at the country level. UNAIDS is leading the way, with its cosponsors and the Secretariat having accepted special responsibility in their respective areas of expertise:

Convening Role of U.N. Agencies for Specific Program Areas

- United Nations Children's Fund (UNICEF): orphans and vulnerable children
- United Nations Development Program (UNDP): governance; development planning

- United Nations Population Fund (UNFPA): condom programming for prevention of HIV; young people
- United Nations Office on Drugs and Crime (UNODC): injecting drug use
- International Labor Organization (ILO): world of work
- United Nations Educational, Scientific and Cultural Organization (UNESCO): education
- World Health Organization (WHO): care and support within the health sector; prevention of HIV transmission to pregnant women, mothers, and children
- World Bank: evaluation of HIV/AIDS programs at country level; economic impact
- Joint United Nations Programme on HIV/AIDS Secretariat: men who have sex with men; commercial sex work; evaluation of HIV/AIDS programming at global level

The idea is not that these agencies are solely responsible for these program areas but, rather, that they have a facilitating (or "convening") role in promoting, supporting, and monitoring the achievement of specific targets. The UNAIDS Secretariat will facilitate key areas not covered by other U.N. organizations (listed above) and provide overall coordination and support to other partners.

Benefits of Monitoring Framework of the Declaration of Commitment on HIV/AIDS

All member states agreed to report back to the U.N. General Assembly on an annual basis on progress made in reaching the declaration's targets. UNAIDS and key partners (including monitoring and evaluation [M&E] practitioners; academics; and representatives from research institutions, donor agencies, and governmental and nongovernmental organizations from member states) developed a monitoring framework and indicators, facilitated through the global Monitoring and Evaluation Reference Group. The purpose of this framework is to help member states to keep track of progress on key elements of the declaration. The declaration indicators become the core national indicators in addition to others that countries select to address country-specific needs.

The framework builds on existing data collection tools and aims to be comprehensive, covering all sectors and all levels of efforts (from inputs at global level to impacts at country level), yet simple in its implementation. There are eighteen core declaration indicators, five at the global and thirteen at the national level. Global-level indicators focus on international partners' commitment through increased resources, policy improvement, and advocacy efforts. National-level indicators cover governments' commitment, HIV/AIDS-related programs in the areas of education, health, labor, orphans' support, youth, injecting-drug users, and impacts (Tables 3.1 and 3.2). The

Table 3.1. Global and National Core Indicators for Declaration Implementation

Level	Indicators	Reporting Schedule	Method of Data Collection
Global Commitment and action	Amount of funds spent by international donors on HIV/AIDS in developing countries and countries in transition	Annual	Survey on financial resource flows
	Amount of public funds available for research and development of vaccines and microbicides	Annual	Survey on financial resource flows
	Percentage of transnational companies that are present in developing countries and that have HIV/AIDS workplace policies and programs	Annual	Desk review
	Percentage of international organizations that have workplace policies and programs	Annual	Desk review
	Assessment of HIV/AIDS advocacy efforts	Annual	Qualitative desk assessment(s)
National Commitment and action	Amount of national funds spent by governments on HIV/AIDS	Biennial	Survey on financial resource flows
	National Composite Policy Index[a]	Biennial	Country assessment Questionnaire
Program and behavior	Percentage of schools with teachers who have been trained in life-skills-based HIV/AIDS education and who taught it during the last academic year	Biennial	School-based survey and education program review
	Percentage of large enterprises or companies that have HIV/AIDS workplace policies and programs	Biennial	Workplace survey

Indicator	Frequency	Data source
Percentage of patients with sexually transmitted infections at health care facilities who are appropriately diagnosed, treated, and counseled	Biennial	Health facility survey
Percentage of HIV-infected pregnant women receiving a complete course of antiretroviral prophylaxis to reduce the risk of mother-to-child transmission	Biennial	Program monitoring and estimates
Percentage of people with advanced HIV infection receiving antiretroviral combination therapy	Biennial	Population-based survey
Percentage of injecting-drug users who have adopted behaviors that reduce transmission of HIV[b]		
Percentage of young people aged 15 to 24 who both correctly identify ways of preventing the sexual transmission of HIV and who reject major misconceptions about HIV transmission[c] Target: 90 percent by 2005; 95 percent by 2010	Every 4 to 5 years	
Percentage of young people aged 15 to 24 reporting the use of a condom during sexual intercourse with a nonregular sexual partner[c]	Every 4 to 5 years	Population-based survey
Ratio of current school attendance among orphans to that among nonorphans, aged 10 to 14[c]	Every 4 to 5 years	Population-based survey
Impact Percentage of young people aged 15 to 24 who are HIV-infected[c] Target: 25 percent in most affected countries by 2005; 25 percent reduction globally by 2010	Biennial	HIV sentinel surveillance
Percentage of HIV-infected infants born to HIV-infected mothers Target: 20 percent reduction by 2005; 50 percent reduction by 2010	Biennial	Estimate based on program coverage

[a]See Table 3.2.
[b]Applicable to countries where injecting-drug use is an established mode of HIV transmission.
[c]Millennium Development Goals.

Table 3.2. National Composite Policy Index

Strategic plan	Country has developed multisectorial strategies to combat HIV/AIDS
	Country has integrated HIV/AIDS into its general development plans
	Country has a functional national multisectorial HIV/AIDS management or coordination body
	Country has a functional national HIV/AIDS body that promotes interaction among government, the private sector, and civil society
	Country has a functional HIV/AIDS body that assists the coordination of civil society organizations
	Country has evaluated the effects of HIV/AIDS on its socioeconomic status for planning purposes
	Country has a strategy that addresses HIV/AIDS issues among its national uniformed services (including armed forces and civil defense forces)
Prevention	Country has a general policy or strategy to promote IEC on HIV/AIDS
	Country has a policy or strategy promoting reproductive and sexual health education for young people
	Country has a policy or strategy that promotes IEC and other health interventions for groups with high or increasing rates of HIV infection
	Country has a policy or strategy that promotes IEC and other health interventions for cross-border migrants
	Country has a policy or strategy to expand access, including among vulnerable groups, to essential preventative commodities
	Country has a policy or strategy to reduce mother-to-child transmission.
Human rights	Country has laws and regulations that protect people living with HIV/AIDS against discrimination
	Country has laws and regulations that protect groups of people identified as being especially vulnerable to HIV/AIDS against discrimination
	Country has a policy to ensure equal access for men and women to prevention and care, with emphasis on vulnerable populations
	Country has a policy to ensure that HIV/AIDS research protocols involving human subjects are reviewed and approved by an ethics committee
Care and support	Country has a policy or strategy to promote comprehensive HIV/AIDS care and support, with emphasis on vulnerable groups
	Country has a policy or strategy to ensure or improve access to HIV/AIDS-related medicines, with emphasis on vulnerable groups
	Country has a policy or strategy to address the additional needs of orphans and other vulnerable children

IEC: Information, Education, Communication

National Action Indicator: Number 2.

Source: Joint United Nations Programme on HIV/AIDS (2002a).

core indicators have been incorporated into a document entitled *Monitoring the Declaration of Commitment on HIV/AIDS: Guidelines on the Construction of Core Indicators,* which provides member states with technical guidance on the methods, tools, and frequency for measuring the indicators in a standardized way (Joint United Nations Programme on HIV/AIDS, 2002a). Throughout the development process, efforts have been made to harmonize the indicators with those of other major initiatives, such as the Millennium Development Goals (United Nations Development Program, 2004), to ensure integration and to minimize the data collection burden on countries.

Are the declaration indicators adding to the current burden of country reporting? It can be argued that most of these indicators should be core to any HIV/AIDS prevention, care, and support program in any country at any stage of its HIV/AIDS epidemic, and as such, they should be part of any national strategic plan. Most of the declaration's indicators are well established because they were drawn from and build on other internationally recommended indicator handbooks (Joint United Nations Programme on HIV/AIDS, 2000). However, some indicators are "new," purposively pushing programs toward an extended response and promoting activities in the private sector, the education system, and in vulnerable groups. Also, some indicators are specific to particular HIV epidemics, such as the indicators related to injecting-drug use. A recent review of national M&E plans revealed that, indeed, most core indicators have been included—although not necessarily measured—and many have been adopted by international agencies and key donors for accountability reporting (Joint United Nations Programme on HIV/AIDS, 2003a).

Implementing the declaration's monitoring framework has proved to be a major challenge but at the same time an opportunity for strengthening national M&E systems. Actions to facilitate the capacity-building process started in 2002 through intensive training of national government officials from the national AIDS commissions and the ministry of health at both regional and national levels (coordinated by the MEASURE Evaluation Project at the University of North Carolina with the participation of bilateral agencies, U.N. system organizations, and academic institutions). Participants developed or reviewed feasible short-term M&E plans and focused on a limited number of relevant and measurable indicators, including the declaration indicators. Other capacity-building efforts consisted of the establishment of several M&E technical resource networks composed of national M&E experts and relevant institutions. Members of these networks were trained to provide technical assistance and on-the-job training to member states in their region.

In addition, the UNAIDS Secretariat provided countries with a user-friendly data management tool, the Country Response Information System, that permits the compilation, analysis, and dissemination of relevant HIV/AIDS information. Under the responsibility of the national AIDS commission, the Country Response Information System will house data obtained on core and additional indicators for use in monitoring the implementation of the Declaration of Commitment on HIV/AIDS (Joint United Nations Programme on HIV/AIDS, 2003b). This system will help validate data and give credibility to national HIV/AIDS indicator reports. Indeed, asking countries to monitor and report on their own progress is a sensitive process and potentially open to reporting bias.

Lessons Learned from the 2003 Declaration Reporting

More than one hundred member states reported on their national response to HIV/AIDS with a focus on the declaration's policy and strategy development targets. The respondent countries represent 95 percent of the estimated global number of cases of HIV infection. In terms of response rate, this is unprecedented in the history of the U.N. system. The national reports were consolidated into a *Progress Report on the Global Response to the HIV/AIDS Epidemic, 2003*, and presented for discussion at UNGASS (Joint United Nations Programme on HIV/AIDS, 2002b, 2003a). (The report is available on the UNAIDS Web site for accountability to constituencies and for stimulating exchange among countries.) This report represents the most comprehensive assessment to date of the state of global, regional, and national responses to HIV/AIDS. The following are a few selected findings:

• International and domestic spending in 2003 amounted to US$4.7 billion in low- and middle-income countries, a 20 percent increase compared with 2002 and a 500 percent increase compared with 1996. However, this is less than half of what will be needed by 2005 and less than one-third of needed amounts in 2007.

• Virtually all heavily affected countries have comprehensive, multisectoral national HIV/AIDS strategies and government-led national bodies to coordinate the response to the epidemic.

• Thirty-eight percent of countries have yet to adopt legislation to prevent discrimination against people living with HIV/AIDS, and only 36 percent of countries have legal measures in place to prohibit discrimination against populations that are especially vulnerable to HIV/AIDS.

• As of December 2002, women accounted for 58 percent of all people living with HIV/AIDS in sub-Saharan Africa. However, nearly one-third of countries lack policies that ensure women's equal access to critical prevention and care services.

• There is extremely low coverage of HIV-prevention services: only a fraction of people at risk of contracting HIV have meaningful access to basic prevention services.

• There is extremely low antiretroviral therapy coverage: whereas an estimated 5 to 6 million people currently need antiretroviral therapy in low- and middle-income countries, only thirty thousand people in these regions were obtaining such therapy as of December 2002.

Table 3.3. Indicator Response Rate for Selected Program Areas

Selected Weakest Areas in Reporting	Countries' Response Rate
School teachers' training in life skills	34/104
Workplace policy	26/104
STD case management	15/104
Prevention of mother to child transmission	26/104
Antiretroviral therapy	26/104
Prevention programs for injecting-drug users	9/20

STD, sexually transmitted disease.

The following challenges to achieving the declaration's targets were most commonly cited: insufficient financial resources to implement and scale up interventions; lack of human resources and technical capacity in many areas of HIV programming, especially at the local level; stigma and discrimination; and weak monitoring and evaluation systems. The last will be discussed below.

Most national reports were prepared by national AIDS councils or equivalent bodies. In two-thirds of the cases, these national bodies sought input from civil society. Three-quarters of the countries stated that these national reports were publicly available. The section on policy indicators was completed by 87 percent of respondent countries, but only 40 percent of countries provided information on key national program and behavioral indicators (see Table 3.3). The level of information requested has proved to be too detailed. For example, even a simple breakdown of indicators by age and sex or urban versus rural domains for some indicators could not be provided, even though these data were available through existing sources such as the World Health Organization (WHO) database on health programs (World Health Organization, 2004) or the Demographic and Health Survey database (MEASURE/Demographic and Health Survey, 2004). It is possible that these data were also available through other line ministries or public institutions such as the Bureau of Statistics, but it seems that the national AIDS councils were either not aware or were not able to obtain data from these other sources. This indicates a need for increased collaboration and coordination because these are essential data to guide strategic planning and monitoring of the national response to HIV/AIDS.

To consolidate validity, UNAIDS reviewed country data presented in the report and compared them with other sources. Apart from policy and behavioral indicators, the quality of reported data was generally poor (Joint United Nations Programme on HIV/AIDS, 2003a). Financial reporting was particularly weak, possibly because of the complexity of capturing national-level expenditures. Validation and comparison between countries was also difficult because of the variation in national financial tracking systems. Also, few countries were able to provide aggregated national service coverage data because of weak health information systems.

In general, countries that received direct support (for example, assistance of consultants, participation in training workshops on M&E) submitted more comprehensive reports with more accurate data because the data had already been discussed and validated to some extent before submission. Countries with strong support from the U.N. theme group—the coordination mechanism for the U.N. system's response to HIV/AIDS in countries—or with strong assistance from the UNAIDS country program advisor also provided reports of better quality. Without this technical and financial support, many countries would likely have not been able to complete their declaration indicator report.

The declaration endorsed by so many governments was an extraordinary opportunity to raise concerns about HIV/AIDS control program implementation and the measurement of program coverage and effectiveness. It is surprising that twenty years after the beginning of such a threatening epidemic, many countries still do not have a basic information system to monitor the day-to-day implementation of their HIV/AIDS programs to ensure that the most effective approaches are being implemented and to provide accountability to communities and donors. Seventy-five percent of respondent countries reported that inadequate M&E capacity was one of the most serious challenges to meet the declaration's targets. This was confirmed by the responses given in the declaration questionnaire on the status of M&E systems: 43 percent of countries reported having an M&E plan, and only 24 percent indicated that they had an M&E budget to carry out M&E activities. Most countries (88 percent) indicated that they had a formal health information system. However, almost half of them did not have such a system operational at the subnational level, making it difficult to obtain standardized national-level program monitoring data because these are generally fed up from the local to the national level.

A more detailed discussion with some national governments on lessons learned from the reporting on the declaration's progress took place from October through December 2003. This confirmed the fact that most countries do not possess the basic elements of a sound M&E system. Countries highlighted four major obstacles: the fact that M&E activities focus on HIV prevalence and behavioral surveillance data, with little effort made on collecting national-level program inputs, activities, and outputs; the nonexistence of a national-level information system that compiles all HIV/AIDS-related data on the HIV epidemic and the national response to it; the lack of or weak coordination mechanisms among the different sectors involved in a multisectoral response to HIV/AIDS; and competing data needs from various donors. In the words of one participant: "An epidemic of indicators has spread, and most international agencies' donors are now infected." As a result, the focus has reportedly not been on using the data for policy and program improvement but rather on reporting for accountability purposes.

Insufficient investment in staff and lack of funds was also pointed out as an issue, although people recognized that funding is now increasing.

Indeed, in many countries, only one or two M&E experts are responsible for coordinating the implementation of the country's M&E plan, and there is generally limited coordination with regions and districts within the country. However, the M&E unit too often perceives its role to be one of implementing or directly supervising implementation of M&E activities, rather than the more appropriate role of coordinating M&E with a range of national ministries and implementing agencies. In addition, no formalized links are established with technical and other resources.

Many discussants also recognized their failure to ensure careful analysis and interpretation of M&E data by integrating data from a range of available data sources such as HIV and sexually transmitted disease surveillance, tuberculosis surveillance, program inputs and outputs, and behavioral data at national and local levels. Brief meetings related to data analysis are usually the rule. However, without sufficient time spent on understanding the true dynamics of the HIV/AIDS epidemic in relation to the national response, national AIDS councils will be unable to plan strategically and improve both programs and M&E systems over time.

Conclusion

The Declaration of Commitment on HIV/AIDS signed by 189 member states of the United Nations in June 2001 has been instrumental in creating a common platform for action, defining core agendas, and clarifying respective roles and responsibilities of all partners. By setting concrete and time-bound targets, the declaration has put pressure on member states to implement and scale up interventions and report on achievements on a regular basis. A comprehensive yet simple monitoring framework was developed to assist countries with progress reporting.

Despite the unprecedented reporting response, with 103 countries submitting a progress report to the 2003 UNGASS, the low response rate for some core indicators and the poor quality of reported data underscore the need to build robust M&E systems anchored within sound data management and use. Such systems are urgently needed to scale up interventions based on evidence. It is hoped that member states and their partners from the U.N. system, the civil society, and the private sector will demonstrate strong leadership in the coming years and live up to their commitments. However, national governments need to drive the entire implementation process from the planning to the reporting stage. This includes a commitment to using the monitoring framework both for learning about successful and less successful programs and for meeting the targets set for 2005 and 2010.

Applying lessons learned from the 2003 declaration reporting, a number of countries have already taken action leading to improved M&E systems. Some countries have committed to strengthen the M&E unit within the national AIDS council for improved coordination of M&E activities. Still others have decided to start using the UNAIDS Country Response Information System to manage and generate strategic information on HIV/AIDS and to train selected local- and national-level people involved in data collection and processing to improve data quality. A large number of them have also set up national M&E reference groups composed of all M&E actors from line ministries, bilateral agencies, U.N. system organizations, and nongovernmental organizations to ensure proper coordination. Countries that received funding from the World Bank and from the Global Fund to Fight AIDS, Tuberculosis and Malaria—both strong advocates of performance-based disbursement—have also invested in a program monitoring system to track inputs, activities, and output data, including quality assurance mechanisms (see Chapter Six, this issue).

To assist countries in this enormous task, UNAIDS and partners have also initiated a number of actions in the area of M&E. UNAIDS will prepare detailed guidelines to assist member states in the preparation of the next declaration report, due in 2006. The core indicators for monitoring implementation of the declaration may need revision. According to comments of national M&E experts, core indicators for important program areas such as indicators f voluntary counseling and testing and blood safety are missing. Other indicators, such as the reduction in the number of casual partners or delaying first sexual intercourse, may require more prominence. Both the specifications and data collection methods for some indicators may also need improvement to increase consistency among countries. In addition to improving the instructions for reporting, the UNAIDS M&E capacity is being expanded through the deployment in 2004 of twenty-four M&E officers at both country and regional levels and through targeted national and regional trainings. These UNAIDS M&E officers and other newly recruited staff in bilateral agencies will play an instrumental role in assisting countries in the coordination of the entire process from planning for to reporting on the declaration. UNAIDS is also spearheading efforts to obtain agreement from key donors to adhere to the "three ones principles" (one national HIV/AIDS action framework, one national AIDS authority, one M&E system), which promotes coordination among donors as well as between donors and national AIDS programs (Joint United Nations Programme on HIV/AIDS, 2004). The main objective of the "three ones" is to enhance effectiveness, timeliness, and sustainability of results, which are urgently required if all stakeholders are serious about meeting the 2005 targets.

In summary, we have learned four key lessons from our experience to date with the implementation and monitoring of the Declaration of Commitment on HIV/AIDS:

- On the one hand, the formal commitment from member states to fight HIV/AIDS brings a renewed sense of urgency and solidarity to the task. This has been instrumental in defining priorities for action linked to concrete and time-bound targets, in clarifying the roles and responsibilities of all actors engaged in the national response to HIV/AIDS, and in pressing national programs to start building robust M&E systems.

• On the other hand, formal commitment cannot be translated into action if not supported by adequate financial, human, and technical resources.

• Indicators can be selected purposively to push programs toward an extended and more comprehensive response to HIV/AIDS and to promote activities in areas not previously covered.

• The fact that people recognize that global and national indicators are critical information in and of itself does not guarantee that the necessary data are feasible to collect, are collected, are valid, and are used. More effort is needed to have a broad-based consultation on and buy-in from actors representing all levels of M&E. In addition, appropriate, timely, and intensive technical support is needed to strengthen the M&E efforts of national and subnational agencies.

The first progress report, which presents data on selected global- and national-level indicators, represents the most comprehensive assessment to date of the state of global, regional, and national responses on the broad range of challenges posed by HIV/AIDS. This is critical information that will enable the objective measurement of progress and ensure that governments and donors alike are held accountable for the results.

References

Joint United Nations Programme on HIV/AIDS. *National AIDS Programs: A Guide to Monitoring and Evaluation.* Geneva: Joint United Nations Programme on HIV/AIDS, 2000.

Joint United Nations Programme on HIV/AIDS. *United Nations General Assembly Special Session Declaration of Commitment on HIV/AIDS.* Geneva: Joint United Nations Programme on HIV/AIDS, 2001.

Joint United Nations Programme on HIV/AIDS. *Monitoring the Declaration of Commitment on HIV/AIDS: Guidelines on Construction of Core Indicators.* Geneva: Joint United Nations Programme on HIV/AIDS, 2002a.

Joint United Nations Programme on HIV/AIDS. *Report of the Secretary-General on Progress Towards Implementation of the Declaration of Commitment on HIV/AIDS.* Geneva: Joint United Nations Programme on HIV/AIDS, 2002b.

Joint United Nations Programme on HIV/AIDS. *Progress Report on the Global Response to the HIV/AIDS Epidemic, 2003: Follow up to the 2001 UNGASS [United Nations General Assembly Special Session] on HIV/AIDS.* Geneva: Joint United Nations Programme on HIV/AIDS, 2003a.

Joint United Nations Programme on HIV/AIDS. *Country Response Information System Manual 2003.* Geneva: Joint United Nations Programme on HIV/AIDS, 2003b.

Joint United Nations Programme on HIV/AIDS. "Three Ones: Principles for the Coordination of National AIDS Responses." 2004. [http://www.unaids.org/en/about+unaids/what+is+unaids/unaids+at+country+level/the+three+ones.asp]. Accessed June 30, 2004.

Joint United Nations Programme on HIV/AIDS, World Health Organization. *Evaluation of a National AIDS Program: A Methods Package—Prevention of HIV Infection.* Geneva: Joint United Nations Programme on HIV/AIDS, 1999.

MEASURE/Demographic and Health Surveys. "HIV/AIDS Survey Indicator Database." 2004. [http://www.measuredhs.com/hivdata]. July 20, 2004.

United Nations Development Program. "Millennium Development Goals." 2004. [http//www.undp.org/mdg]. Accessed June 30, 2004.

World Health Organization. "The HealthMapper." Communicable Disease Surveillance and Response (CSR). 2004.[http://www.who.int/csr/mapping/tools/healthmapper/healthmapper/en]. Accessed Feb. 10, 2004.

NICOLE MASSOUD *is a monitoring and evaluation adviser at the Joint United Nations Programme on HIV/AIDS Secretariat, based in Geneva, Switzerland.*

PAUL DE LAY *is the director of Monitoring and Evaluation for the Joint UN Programme on HIV/AIDS, based in Geneva, Switzerland.*

MICHEL CARAEL *retired from the chief evaluation position in the Joint United Nations Programme on HIV/AIDS in 2004 and is currently a professor at the Free University of Brussels, Belgium, and consultant in evaluation.*

4

In building on each agency's strengths, we must identify incentives and opportunities for collaboration, with the fundamental consensus that working together in a harmonized manner is better than going it alone.

Efforts in Collaboration and Coordination of HIV/AIDS Monitoring and Evaluation: Contributions and Lessons of Two U.S. Government Agencies in a Global Partnership

Deborah Rugg, John Novak, Greet Peersman, Karen A. Heckert, Jack Spencer, Katherine Marconi

Collaborative partnerships have become more common in public health in recent years, operating at local, national, and international levels (El Ansari, Phillips, and Hammick, 2001). These partnerships involve multiple stakeholders addressing a range of health issues, such as reproductive health, substance abuse, and sexually transmitted diseases including human immunodeficiency virus and acquired immunodeficiency syndrome (HIV/AIDS) (for comprehensive reviews, see Israel, Schulz, Parker, and Becker, 1998; Roussos and Fawcett, 2000; El Ansari, Phillips, and Hammick, 2001). The results of this approach in improving health outcomes at the community level are mixed, mainly due to difficulty in attributing the effects to the partnership and documenting the process. From the literature, it appears that evaluating the role of collaborative efforts at national and international levels is even more challenging, and although there are some, there have not been many successful attempts (Milstein and Kreuter, 2000; Roussos and Fawcett, 2000). Despite the lack of rigorous evaluations, some of the factors associated with successful international partnerships have been identified. Such factors include knowledge of host-country resources, personal contacts with key local partners, knowledge of the international environments, and having country government support for joint projects. Factors that limit success

NEW DIRECTIONS FOR EVALUATION, no. 103, Fall 2004 © Wiley Periodicals, Inc.

include, but are not limited to, conflicts of interest—either real or apparent—and the additional time that is required for multiagency negotiations and implementation. For any collaborative effort or partnership to be successful, some factors are essential: a clear purpose, defined contributions of each partner, activities that are in line with country government guidelines, and a defined management and implementation plan (Root, 1994). In this chapter, we seek to contribute to the discussion about collaborative partnerships at the national and international levels by presenting the experience of two U.S. government bilateral agencies—the U.S. Agency for International Development (USAID) and the Centers for Disease Control and Prevention (CDC), which have now partnered with other U.S. government agencies to implement the President's Emergency Plan for AIDS Relief. The experiences from other major international multilateral agencies such as the Joint United Nations Programme on HIV/AIDS (UNAIDS), the World Health Organization (WHO), and the World Bank, while introduced as part of the global monitoring and evaluation (M&E) partnership, are discussed elsewhere in this issue.

Because the AIDS pandemic respects no national boundaries, the global community has become involved in providing the financial and technical resources necessary to prevent the further spread of HIV and, more recently, to offer care and treatment services to those already infected. Over the past few years, the U.S. government, the World Bank, the Global Fund to Fight AIDS, Tuberculosis and Malaria (Global Fund), and other donors have dramatically increased their funding for HIV/AIDS programs around the world, committing over $20 billion. For example, in 2003, the U.S. Congress passed the President's Emergency Plan for AIDS Relief and appropriated, as part of the 2004 budget, $2.4 billion to the emergency plan. All U.S. government agency international HIV/AIDS programs now jointly use a single, coordinated global HIV/AIDS strategy. With this has come the commensurate demand for M&E to ensure accountability, measure program progress and success, inform necessary programmatic changes, and direct funding to achieve maximum effect. Given the numerous stakeholders involved in the global fight against HIV/AIDS, coordination and collaboration are essential. No single agency alone can adequately respond to the growing need for M&E data. Moreover, as the information needs of donors, national AIDS programs, and local governments significantly overlap, common sense tells us that all agencies must take concerted action to reduce the redundancy, competition, and fragmentation of M&E activities at the country level. Successful partnerships will enhance the ability of all stakeholders to achieve their common goal of attaining sound data in a timely manner.

Recognizing the growing need for coordination, all major multilateral and bilateral organizations and many national governments recently endorsed the "commitment to concerted action" statement (Joint United Nations Programme on HIV/AIDS, 2004). This international call to action focuses on country-level coordination and articulates three unifying principles to guide implementation of AIDS programming at the country level. The "three ones principle" calls for *one* organizing authority in country that all donors work with; *one* national strategic plan that all donors use to plan their activities; and *one* comprehensive national M&E plan that all donors work to support, including collecting data, developing national databases, and building the national M&E capacity (Joint United Nations Programme on HIV/AIDS, 2004).

In this chapter, we first highlight the experiences in global M&E coordination and collaboration. We then describe the collaboration experiences of two U.S. government agencies active in HIV prevention and care, USAID and CDC, and how they have participated in the global M&E partnership to set international standards and provide direct M&E support to national AIDS programs. As the main U.S. development agency, USAID works generally through country and regional missions to implement multisector programs, including preventive health and related services, through non-governmental organizations. The CDC is the main U.S public health agency and part of the U.S. Department of Health and Human Services (DHHS), working both domestically and internationally. The CDC's international HIV/AIDS efforts operate generally through field offices that support the ministries' of health and their implementing partners. The CDC and USAID agencies have been working together intensively on HIV/AIDS M&E since 1999 and coordinating M&E financial and technical support to countries around the world. In 2004 they joined other U.S. government agencies in formulating one strategy for international HIV monitoring and evaluation. In fifteen HIV/AIDS focus countries, the agencies participate in a mission team that submits a yearly HIV/AIDS operational plan.

We discuss the challenges faced and the successes achieved in harmonizing M&E strategies between our two agencies. We then describe the application of our M&E approaches within a real-life context in Cambodia, highlighting how our agencies work together on the ground to support the work of ministries of health, multisectoral national HIV/AIDS programs and councils, and a range of other governmental and nongovernmental organizations to strengthen implementation of M&E systems. It is important to note that other chapters in this issue highlight the collaborative work of other agencies as well, such as UNAIDS (Chapter Three), WHO (Chapter Five), and the World Bank (Chapter Six). To conclude, we call for enhanced coordination among *all* in-country partners within the commitment to the "three ones principle."

Global Monitoring and Evaluation Partnership

The ultimate success of the global fight against HIV/AIDS will depend on the scale, scope, and quality of the prevention, care, and treatment programs delivered in each of the affected countries. Conducting M&E activities is paramount because they provide important data on program progress, allow for better program management and accountability, and provide data to plan strategically for future resource needs. With limited M&E resources and overlapping data needs, collaboration and coordination between agencies and with governments has mutual benefits. These opportunities for synergy, however, need to be actively sought and nurtured to achieve the best use of available resources.

The multiagency M&E logic model (Figure 2.1) is a valuable tool for depicting how each agency's program contributes to reaching a common goal (for example, reduced incidence of HIV transmission) within a national AIDS program. It illustrates that whereas outputs, the direct products or deliverables of activities, may be traced back to agency-specific support, the expected outcomes of programs supported by different agencies usually overlap, and long-term effects result from the entire HIV/AIDS program in the country. Although it is important for individual agencies to monitor their program outputs, it is difficult, and indeed unnecessary, to measure the relative contribution from each agency to the impact on the epidemic. Instead, the effect of the consolidated national response to HIV/AIDS or the collective effectiveness is best monitored through disease surveillance and population-based surveys that measure trends in risk-taking behaviors and other factors (such as quality of life). Chapter Two in this issue provides more detail on the kinds of information needed at each level.

In 1999, recognizing the benefits of a unified approach to M&E at the national level, UNAIDS reestablished the M&E Reference Group, which includes UNAIDS, the United Nations Children's Fund (UNICEF), WHO, the World Bank, the Global Fund, and two U.S. government agencies: the CDC and USAID, among other key global partners. A subset of this group, mainly the agencies most active in M&E listed above, formed an informal global M&E partnership that has evolved and is still operating today. It was envisaged that the review and endorsement of common M&E approaches and tools by all participating members would pave the way for a simplified and coordinated effort. With the wide range of indicators and data collection instruments to evaluate the success of HIV/AIDS programs already available, M&E specialists from around the world were brought together to summarize the best M&E practices at the national program level and to recommend options to improve national M&E systems. This was a significant challenge because many agencies were already committed to and had implemented their own M&E strategies, paradigms, indicators, and tools. After several consultation meetings and much discussion, it became clear, however, that it was in everyone's best interest to support a common simple framework and collaborative approach. Competing agency strategies would foster redundancy and confusion at the country level and create demands that were far too complex to be sustainable. This situation would clearly undermine the ability of national governments to establish strong M&E systems, which all agencies need to rely on for their data requirements. As a result, the M&E Reference Group agreed to use the basic input-activities-output-outcome-impact monitoring framework

Figure 4.1. Multiagency Monitoring and Evaluation Logic Model]

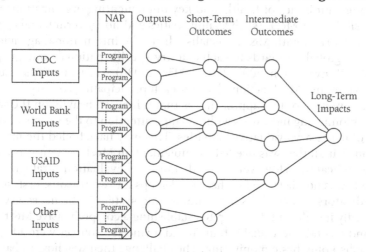

Source: Adapted from Milstein and Kreuter (2000).

(see Chapter Two, this issue) and to develop a simple harmonized set of indicators for use at the country level. To obtain endorsement, national AIDS program managers from various countries were involved in the development process and in conducting several field tests for feasibility and utility of the new indicators. It took about two years for all participating agencies to produce, test, and endorse the standardized international indicators. UNAIDS, then, with the financial and technical support from USAID (through the Measure and Evaluation to Assess and Use Results [MEASURE] Project), WHO, UNICEF, the World Bank, CDC's Global AIDS Program, and others, published the landmark guidance document entitled *National AIDS Programs: A Guide to Monitoring and Evaluation* (Joint United Nations Programme on HIV/AIDS, 2000) (referred to as UNAIDS Guide to M&E in this chapter). This document became widely endorsed as the international standard for HIV/AIDS M&E.

However, the joint issues of country-level endorsement and the national capacity to implement the guidance were still problematic. To address these issues, a series of regional M&E capacity-building workshops were designed to discuss the new indicators in the context of each country's specific situation and to address how to develop a comprehensive national M&E plan, including internal and external resources for implementation. UNAIDS, USAID, the CDC, WHO, and the World Bank co-organized and co-facilitated this series of four regional M&E workshops: in Entebbe, Uganda (April 2001), where seven African countries participated; in Dakar, Senegal (February 2002), where seventeen additional African countries participated; in Bangkok, Thailand (November 2003), where five Asian countries participated; and in Kiev, Ukraine (December 2003), where twelve eastern

European countries participated. Representatives from the national AIDS programs, ministries of health, and key implementing organizations with responsibility for M&E (such as universities and nongovernmental organizations) worked with M&E specialists from the international agencies to apply the global standards to each country-specific national strategic plan (MEASURE Evaluation, 2001, 2002, 2003a, 2003b). The workshops resulted in twelve-month M&E action plans for each participating country.

A limitation of this approach was that it focused heavily on the selection of monitoring indicators without equal attention to the variety of other types of necessary evaluative activities. This may have fueled the misconception that all that was needed to implement an M&E system was monitoring indicators. However, the full range of evaluation strategies and methods was not discussed in these workshops for two reasons: first, selecting indicators and establishing a monitoring system is the necessary, but admittedly insufficient, first step to establishing a comprehensive M&E system, and second, the available human and financial resources were adequate to establish only basic monitoring. The challenge then was how to balance the need to establish monitoring systems with the need to support priority evaluations and operationalize to implement these strategies with sufficient funding. Without a coordinated plan for evaluation activities, information about what is and is not working and how to improve programs in the specific country context was addressed on an ad hoc basis, if at all, compromising the ability to answer key questions and design effective programs. While support for solid program evaluation and a comprehensive M&E plan was the long-range intention of the global M&E partnership, it has taken longer than expected to build the capacity to conduct more than basic monitoring.

Another challenge has been that, whereas donors felt that the standards set out in the UNAIDS Guide to M&E were clear and that the process of making them relevant to each country was straightforward, this was not always the case. In addition, the individuals attending the meetings were not always the right audience; that is, they were not necessarily the individuals who could make decisions about the national M&E systems, were not adequately knowledgeable about the national plan, or did not have any M&E role or responsibility. So the country action plans for M&E developed during the workshops still needed wider endorsement in each country, which did not always happen. This clearly affected some countries' ability to implement the short-term M&E action plans.

A follow-up meeting with representatives from nineteen African countries in October 2003 in Dakar assessed the progress made in M&E implementation. The following main lessons were learned and recommendations made for improving M&E at the national level:

- Local M&E capacity and interest in training were seriously lacking
- Dedicated and trained staff were needed for M&E and ideally a specific M&E unit located in the national AIDS program

- A strong leader or director with technical and managerial skills was needed for M&E
- There needed to be a dedicated M&E budget with the M&E director having decision-making authority
- There needed to be enhanced ownership of the M&E process and understanding of M&E for program improvement purposes
- A country-level M&E coordination committee or work group was needed to foster concerted action in support of a single national M&E plan (the third "one" in the UNAIDS' "three ones principle")
- A balance was needed between the information demands of the international donors and the needs of the national program

These findings have focused the global M&E partnership on balancing their need for short-term program information with funding to intensify overall national M&E system development and capacity-building efforts. This will require more than formal trainings and hands-on workshops for country personnel and will include identifying and supporting additional staff with M&E expertise to be placed in country-level offices to strengthen national M&E systems. Targeted and timely technical assistance in response to country-identified M&E needs will also be enhanced. In addition to the lessons learned in collaboration at the global level, the U.S. government has made a substantial effort to establish a unified M&E approach across its agencies. Experiences and lessons learned in collaborating and coordinating our response at the headquarters and field levels are discussed next.

Making USAID and CDC Headquarters' Collaboration Work

As discussed earlier, the sum total of all agencies' efforts will determine the effects on the global AIDS epidemic. Building on each agency's strengths and experiences, we must identify incentives and opportunities for collaboration, with the fundamental consensus that working together in a harmonized manner is better than "going it alone." Thus, to establish a successful partnership that fosters effective communications, coordination, and collaboration, the CDC and USAID undertook a range of activities. These included jointly funded, co-organized, and co-facilitated events, some of them with other global partners and some intensively focused on collaboration between the two agencies. As the literature on enhancing interagency collaboration suggests, and as we also experienced, it is crucial to start out a partnership with a basic understanding of the other partner's comparative advantages and an attitude valuing the differences (Fox, 1995; Reed and Collins, 1994; Myrick, forthcoming).

The CDC, a public health agency, and USAID, an international development agency, first had to come together to identify common goals and a common language regarding M&E. This was not an easy task because the two agencies have different institutional affiliations, implementing partners, programmatic emphases, areas of technical expertise, political constraints, and M&E strategies. The first step was for the two agencies headquarters' staff to work together in many meetings to understand these differences and to discuss a common goal, terminology, framework, and unified approach combining public health and development best practices. This required developing a joint strategic vision, negotiating and communicating this vision effectively to bring together all stakeholders, and negotiating consensus and consciously managing the process to achieve results. As the literature on participatory approaches suggests (for example, Picciotto, 1992), building multiagency consensus must involve a meaningful participatory process that includes all stakeholders. Furthermore, the leaders of this process must have faith in a participatory approach.

The next step was getting to know each other's organization, operational procedures, and "corporate culture." Although we initially thought this would be simple, we found it to be an ongoing task that took substantial effort. Several activities became essential. To establish mutual trust, transparency, and effective communications, the CDC and USAID staff conducted the following:

- Agency visits
- Biweekly conference calls
- Quarterly meetings
- Review of agency-specific guidance and cosigned letters of concurrence on major issues
- Activities to foster staff collaboration and interaction with other parts of the agencies (for example, participation in interagency working groups)

Such activities proved critical in maintaining our trust and commitment to the partnership as we experienced the challenge of new agency staff becoming involved, disagreements on technical issues and process, and significant external course-changing events that occurred over which we had little control.

The relationship was further solidified through the mutual experience of joint achievements:

- Joint efforts to organize and conduct M&E workshops and trainings were felt to be more effective than conducting them separately and resulted in further M&E partnerships.
- Joint development of core indicators, joint plans for data collection, and the development of several joint standardized M&E guidance documents provided a common shared experience that fostered a sense of mutual support for a collaborative approach and a coordinated plan. This fostered a strong sense of working toward the same goal and of basically being on the same team.

• Joint global events (such as the capacity-building workshops discussed above) and jointly signed letters of endorsement and invitation gave each agency the sense of equal decision-making authority in the partnership.

• Jointly funded projects at both central and country levels gave agency staff the experience of working together on important tasks, which allowed each to see relevant strengths and contributions.

Written, mutually agreed on, and specific operational plans that allowed for a clear delineation of expectations regarding roles, responsibilities, relationships, timelines, and accountability to the partnership were an important contributor to the joint success of major activities.

A recent important activity of this M&E partnership is the coordination of M&E trainings and technical assistance as part of the new U.S. government global effort. Spearheaded by the CDC with USAID support, the M&E Trainers' Network is composed of all U.S. government international M&E training providers. During 2003, the network developed an M&E training calendar that includes all trainings sponsored by the CDC and USAID and an M&E training participant database that includes key information on all HIV/AIDS M&E trainings sponsored by the U.S. government. These included training type, location, and participant information. This network was later expanded to include all United Nations agencies' HIV/AIDS M&E trainers at a meeting of the UNAIDS M&E Reference Group Subcommittee on M&E Training Harmonization in February 2004 in Divonne, France. Similarly, USAID has spearheaded development of a database and listserv to coordinate these providers' M&E technical assistance to countries. The efforts to coordinate international M&E trainings and technical assistance struggled at first, largely because of overambitious expectations. When these were scaled back and specific achievable targets and resources were set and endorsed by all partners, significant progress was made.

In 2004, USAID and the CDC began to implement joint planning and budgeting for their HIV/AIDS M&E activities with other DHHS agencies, including the Health Resources and Services Administration, and the Peace Corps, U.S. Census Bureau, and the U.S. Department of Defense. This planning and budgeting are part of the coordination led by the newly created Office of the U. S. Global AIDS Coordinator. A series of interagency strategic information working groups have formed to assure continued common approaches to measurement and country M&E support by U.S. government agencies. Whereas the initial focus was on fifteen countries affected by HIV, the U.S. Global AIDS Coordinator oversees and directs all U.S. government international HIV/AIDS activities. The lessons learned by USAID and the CDC in their M&E partnerships form the basis for this effort.

The collaboration on M&E between the U.S. government and its global partners—UNAIDS, WHO, UNICEF, the World Bank, the Global

Fund, and others—has also set in motion an important international partnership. However, we have learned that successful interagency collaboration does not come automatically; it requires substantial effort, good will, trust, and transparency. It also requires setting realistic expectations and seeing a balance between what is contributed and what is gained from the partnership. In addition, we have learned that to sustain the initial enthusiasm, collaboration takes managerial time, appropriate human and fiscal resources, and creativity. Each agency needed to understand the other agency's internal M&E systems, program management, and accountability requirements and constraints. The best way to do this was by working together, not only at the central level, but also at the country level. Thus, the M&E approaches and systems of the U.S. government are highlighted in the country examples given below. Other chapters in this volume (Chapters Three, Five, and Six) describe the collaborative work of others such as UNAIDS, WHO, and the World Bank.

A Country Level Example: Cambodia

Because of its significant HIV/AIDS epidemic and lack of sufficient resources to combat it, Cambodia has received an increase in financial and technical support from both USAID and the CDC over the past few years. A Three-Year Public Health Interim Strategy and an HIV/AIDS Strategic Plan for 2002 to 2005 were developed simultaneously. Core indicators were selected from the *USAID Expanded Response* guidance (U.S. Agency for International Development, 2002), the *Global AIDS Program Indicators Guide* (Centers for Disease Control and Prevention, 2003), and the indicators in the *National AIDS Programs: Guide to Monitoring and Evaluation* produced by the global partnership (Joint United Nations Programme on HIV/AIDS, 2000). Because agreement on international standard indicators and their definitions had already been reached by the U.S. government and others in the global M&E partnership, a solid basis existed for country discussions, which saved considerable time. Adaptation of existing international indicators to the Cambodian context was easier than developing new indicators altogether. The issue was then to see whether there were any gaps, establish appropriate targets, develop estimates, identify data sources, and ensure that high data quality could be achieved. This was done through a consultative process with implementing partners and multiple stakeholders, including the CDC, the USAID Office of HIV/AIDS/Washington, and the National Center for HIV/AIDS, Dermatology, and Sexually Transmitted Infections (NCHADS), part of the Cambodia Ministry of Health. The aim was to provide reliable and valid data to measure changes in national and provincial trends and, at the same time, evaluate U.S. government-supported efforts. Because the CDC and USAID had worked together at the global level, most of the core indicators served both purposes. This provides an explicit example of how global standards can reduce the burden of data collection at the country level. The Cambodian experience also provides an example of how each agency contributes based on its respective expertise and comparative advantage.

For example, in 2003, the CDC worked closely with the Cambodia Office of Public Health, NCHADS, and implementing partners to strengthen the implementation of the ninth round of the HIV Surveillance Survey. This included several important changes to the protocol that included new safeguards to confidentiality (surveillance staff signed an assurance of confidentiality for the first time), development of an informed consent script and a requirement that the consent be documented, decentralization of testing, a switch to the use of rapid-testing technology with commensurate regional training sessions for laboratory staff, and a quality assurance protocol. These changes assured a better, more reliable result compared with previous HIV Surveillance Survey data.

Through a cooperative agreement between the CDC and the University of California at San Francisco, a resident M&E advisor was assigned to establish systems for monitoring the process and outcomes of a province-wide demonstration project in Banteay Mean Chey Province. Staff developed an M&E strategy for this project that aimed to link and coordinate the major HIV prevention and care strategies under one management. A survey integrating HIV and sexually transmitted diseases results with a behavioral questionnaire was created to inform program decisions. If this demonstration project proves to be successful, it will then be replicated in other provinces.

The single most significant collaborative effort in Cambodia between USAID and the CDC took place in mid-2003 in response to the Cambodian government's request to conduct a midterm assessment of the *Ministry of Health's Strategic Plan for HIV/AIDS and STDs Prevention and Care in Cambodia, 2001–2005* (Cambodia Ministry of Health, 2002a). The CDC and USAID representatives co-led the assessment team, which comprised nineteen technical people from NCHADS, the CDC, USAID, UNAIDS, WHO, and the United Kingdom Department for International Development. The core objectives were as follows:

- Review progress toward accomplishing objectives outlined in each of the program areas in the HIV/AIDS Strategic Plan
- Develop recommendations for strengthening the program areas and strategic plan
- Recommend indicators for each of the program areas
- Develop a national HIV/AIDS M&E framework

Approximately thirty additional in-country stakeholders were consulted for initial guidance, contributions throughout the process, and discussion of the preliminary results and recommendations.

The recommendations of this review are the foundation for a revised national strategic plan for 2003 to 2007 (Cambodia Ministry of Health,

2002b) and thus will significantly refocus the HIV/AIDS prevention and care program in Cambodia over the next five years. The government adopted the proposed M&E framework and indicators. The CDC and USAID then worked to further specify the targets and baseline data for each indicator for the years ahead.

An additional example of collaboration and an early example of the "three ones principle," specifically the third component—a single national M&E plan and coordinating committee—is the National HIV/AIDS M&E Coordination Committee that was established with the Ministry of Health and NCHADS, the multisectoral National AIDS Association, nongovernmental organizations, the Global Fund, UNAIDS, and donor partners. This committee is responsible for building consensus on core indicators for each programmatic area; coordinating data collection, analysis, and interpretation; and managing data dissemination and use for central, provincial, and donor-level planning and reporting. The Cambodia Country Team, with representation from NCHADS, participated in the multiagency workshop for strengthening national M&E in Bangkok in November 2003 (mentioned above). Technical assistance for national M&E in Cambodia continues to be provided by the U.S. government.

This country example gives an idea of some of the M&E activities that the U.S. government is supporting through funding and technical assistance. Such support draws on the efforts of the global M&E partnership that provided frameworks and standards and that were then adapted to the country-specific program context and adopted by both the national government and donor agencies, thereby decreasing the burden of data collection on the country. The existence of global standards also facilitated the work of the team assessing the national strategic plan, the results of which directly guided the next strategic planning process and informed the establishment of a coordinating committee for M&E. Looking at specific USAID and CDC inputs, each agency has drawn on its particular strengths: the CDC on its expertise in surveillance and USAID on its expertise with population-based surveys. Both contribute key elements of a national M&E system and make for the efficient use of donor resources. Recognizing that in-country M&E capacity is a major challenge, the CDC also supports a resident M&E advisor.

Conclusion

Although various programmatic responses have not always been well coordinated, the international professional M&E community and its respective agencies have stated that it is imperative that a collaborative approach to M&E is taken at the international level and that activities be coordinated at the country level. Therefore, all major stakeholders at the international level adopted a unified approach to M&E as the first step. The next step is for this global-level commitment to be translated into concrete country-level coordination and collaboration. Although important progress has been made, there is clearly room for improvement. There needs to be intensified coordination of technical support in response to specific country needs. We have found that there is no short cut to achieving comprehensive, sustainable M&E systems and that no single agency can do it alone. We need to be committed to this partnership for the long haul.

In terms of the future, there is an urgent need for more attention to strengthening the capacity for M&E at levels below the national level—provincial, district, and community—including meaningful participation from members of the affected communities. This focus is only just beginning but must rapidly scale up. The international community understandably first focused its attention on establishing a foundation for global and national M&E to provide a basis for justifying further funding. But now it is becoming increasingly clear that national-level data rely on the capacity to collect valid and appropriate data at subnational levels and that the ability to use data for program improvement at the local level is essential. Strengthening this area will also benefit from a collaborative and coordinated approach.

Although collaborations can be both challenging and rewarding, it is important to work proactively on developing and maintaining the partnership, applying the lessons mentioned above, and "staying the course" as jointly charted by all agencies involved. Only then will it be possible to reach the stage where data and other information that have been jointly planned for, funded, and collected are actually used strategically for the clear mutual benefit of multiple agencies and for the betterment of global and national HIV/AIDS policies and programs.

Since the beginning of the AIDS epidemic, one thing that has remained constant has been the dynamic nature and rate of change, both in the epidemic itself and in the subsequent global public health response. Thus, those who embrace a collaborative approach to M&E need to be cognizant of and prepared for the inevitable change in course that is inherent in disease epidemics and the responses to them. The real challenge, however, is to remain flexible and to embrace and incorporate change while maintaining the hard-won standards and accomplishments. It is only in the collective effort that partnerships represent that we can successfully navigate the exciting yet challenging changes and keep our eye on the ultimate goal: that M&E data are collected to help improve programs and target limited resources as effectively as possible.

References

Cambodia Ministry of Health. *Strategic Plan for HIV/AIDS and STDs Prevention and Care in Cambodia, 2001–2005.* Phnom Penh: Ministry of Health, 2002a.

Cambodia Ministry of Health. *Health Sector Strategic Plan 2003–2007.* Phnom Penh: Ministry of Health, 2002b.

Centers for Disease Control and Prevention. *Global AIDS Program Indicators Guide.* Atlanta: Global AIDS Program, Centers for Disease Control and Prevention, 2003.

El Ansari, W., Phillips, C., and Hammick, M. "Collaboration and Partnerships: Developing the Evidence Base." *Health and Social Care in the Community*, 2001, *9*(4), 215–227.

Fox, J. "Collaborative Research Pitfalls Examined: Ethics Colloquium Outlines Key Issues Researchers Need to Consider When Embarking on Collaborative Enterprises." *American Society for Microbiology News*, 1995, *61*, 517–519.

Israel, B., Schulz, A., Parker, E., and Becker, A. "Review of Community-Based Research: Assessing Partnership Approaches to Improve Public Health." *Annual Review in Public Health*, 1998, *19*, 173–202.

Joint United Nations Programme on HIV/AIDS. *National AIDS Programs: A Guide to Monitoring and Evaluation.* Geneva: Joint United Nations Programme on HIV/AIDS, 2000.

Joint United Nations Programme on HIV/AIDS. "Commitment to Principles for Concerted AIDS Action at Country Level." 2004. [http://www.unaids.org/NetTools/Misc/DocInfo.aspx?href=http%3A%2F%2Fgva%2Ddoc%2Dowl%2FWEBcontent%2FDocuments%2Fpub%2FUNA%2Ddocs%2FThree%2DOnes%5FCommitment%5Fen%2Epdf]. Retrieved June 23, 2004. Retrieved June 23, 2004.

MEASURE Evaluation. *Strengthening Monitoring and Evaluation of National AIDS Programs in the Context of the Expanded Response.* Workshop summary, Entebbe, Uganda, Apr. 2001, Chapel Hill, N.C.: MEASURE Evaluation, 2001.

MEASURE Evaluation. *Strengthening Monitoring and Evaluation of National AIDS Programs in the Context of the Expanded Response.* Workshop summary, Dakar, Senegal, Feb. 2002. Chapel Hill, N.C.: MEASURE Evaluation, 2002.

MEASURE Evaluation. *Strengthening Monitoring and Evaluation of National AIDS Programs in the Context of the Expanded Response.* Workshop summary, Dakar, Senegal, Oct. 2003. Chapel Hill, N. C.: MEASURE Evaluation, 2003a.

MEASURE Evaluation. *Strengthening Monitoring and Evaluation of National AIDS Programs in the Context of the Expanded Response.* Workshop summary, Bangkok, Thailand, Nov. 2003. Chapel Hill, N.C.: MEASURE Evaluation, 2003b.

Milstein, B., and Kreuter, M. *A Summary of Logic Models: What Are They and What Can They Do for Planning and Evaluation?* Atlanta: Centers for Disease Control and Prevention, 2000.

Myrick, R. "Experiences in Fostering Agency Collaboration and a Participatory Approach for HIV/AIDS Prevention." *AIDS Education and Prevention,* forthcoming.

Picciotto, R. "Participatory Development: Myths and Dilemmas." World Bank Policy Research Working Paper. Washington, D.C.: World Bank, 1992.

Reed, G. M., and Collins, B. E. "Mental Health Research and Service Delivery: A Three Communities Model." *Psychosocial Rehabilitation Journal,* 1994, *17*, 70–81.

Root, F. R. *Entry Strategies into International Markets.* San Francisco: Jossey-Bass, 1994.

Roussos, S., and Fawcett, S. "A Review of Collaborative Partnerships as a Strategy for Improving Community Health." *Annual Review in Public Health,* 2000, *21*, 369–402.

U.S. Agency for International Development. *USAID Expanded Response.* Washington, D.C.: U.S. Agency for International Development, 2002.

DEBORAH RUGG is the associate director of the Monitoring and Evaluation Team for the Global AIDS Program at the U.S. Centers for Disease Control and Prevention, Atlanta, Georgia.

JOHN NOVAK is the monitoring and evaluation adviser to the U.S. Agency for International Development, Washington D.C.

GREET PEERSMAN is the technical deputy director of the Monitoring and Evaluation Team for the Global AIDS Program at the U.S. Centers for Disease Control and Prevention, Atlanta, Georgia.

KAREN A. HECKERT is the senior adviser for integrating family planning, maternal and child health, and prenatal mother-to-child transmission for the USAID/Regional HIV/AIDS Program for Southern Africa based in Pretoria, South Africa, and formerly was the senior monitoring and evaluation adviser, USAID/Cambodia.

JACK SPENCER is the chief of the CDC Global AIDS Program in Cambodia.

KATHERINE MARCONI is director of strategic information and evaluation in the Office of the U.S. Global AIDS Coordinator, Washington D.C.

5

*National program managers need data from different
geographical areas within the country to plan for and
monitor improvements in service coverage and capacity
for care and treatment of patients with HIV/AIDS. They
need to ensure equitable access to services by those in
need.*

Developing and Implementing Monitoring and Evaluation Methods in the New Era of Expanded Care and Treatment of HIV/AIDS

R. Cameron Wolf, George Bicego, Katherine Marconi,
Ruth Bessinger, Eric van Praag, Shanti Noriega-
Minichiello, Gregory Pappas, Nancy Fronczak,
Greet Peersman, Renée K. Fiorentino, Deborah Rugg,
John Novak

The magnitude of the human immunodeficiency virus and acquired immunodeficiency syndrome (HIV/AIDS) pandemic makes it one of the greatest challenges of our time. Worldwide, over 40 million people are now infected, 95 percent of them in developing countries, and each day this total increases by fourteen thousand (World Health Organization, 2003a). In two decades, the pandemic has claimed nearly 30 million lives (World Health Organization, 2003a), imposing a huge burden on the health infrastructure while threatening progress in development. In sub-Saharan Africa, the most severely affected region of the world, more than 60 percent of hospital beds are occupied by persons with HIV-related disease (De Lay, Ernberg, and Stanecki, 2001). HIV/AIDS has affected not only the health sector but every aspect of human society, undermining the economic, social, and political gains of the past half-century (World Health Organization, 2003a). AIDS has orphaned more than 13 million children, leaving families and communities, often overburdened themselves with AIDS, to care for them (World Health Organization, 2003a). The greatest burdens of disease are concentrated in developing countries.

NEW DIRECTIONS FOR EVALUATION, no. 103, Fall 2004 © Wiley Periodicals, Inc.

The sharp rise in the HIV/AIDS burden worldwide has elicited calls for increased efforts to combat the spread and impact of HIV/AIDS. Efforts must continue with the aim to decrease new infections. At the same time, care and treatment services for those already infected can lead to longer, productive lives, thereby minimizing negative effects on families, communities, and societies at large. Although there is currently no cure for HIV infection, sustained use of combination antiretroviral therapy has been shown to increase survival, improve quality of life, reduce hospitalization and morbidity, and mitigate the socioeconomic effects of HIV/AIDS (World Health Organization, 2004a). Provision of antiretroviral therapy and supportive care has also been associated with decreased stigma and fear (World Health Organization, 2004a). However, of the 6 million people who urgently need antiretroviral therapy in developing countries, fewer than 8 percent are currently receiving it (World Health Organization, 2003a). Increased funding for HIV/AIDS efforts and increased access to affordable drug regimens has been an area of notable advocacy, and the provision of antiretroviral therapy is now becoming a reality in resource-poor settings.

The first United Nations General Assembly Special Session (UNGASS) on HIV/AIDS was held in 2001, resulting in an increased commitment from 189 countries to addressing HIV/AIDS. Under the leadership of the Director General of the United Nations, the Global Fund to Fight AIDS, Tuberculosis and Malaria (Global Fund) was established and has since received pledges in the amount of billions of U.S. dollars from around the globe (see Chapter Three, this issue). The World Bank also sharply increased funding for HIV/AIDS, including provision of grants rather than loans. In 2003, the U.S. government pledged US$15 billion toward AIDS over five years, including a focus on treating 2 million people with antiretroviral therapy and providing care for 10 million people in the highest prevalence countries of Africa and the Caribbean region. At the same time, the World Health Organization (WHO) and its partners launched the "Treat 3 Million by 2005" Initiative as a necessary, achievable target on the way to the ultimate goal of universal access to antiretroviral therapy for everyone who requires such therapy (World Health Organization, 2003a). Because immediate action is required to avert millions of needless deaths, the HIV/AIDS treatment emergency requires strong leadership and partnerships for sustained country support.

Access to antiretroviral therapy is only one component of comprehensive care for HIV/AIDS. People living with HIV/AIDS require a wide range of services, including clinical, psychosocial, economic, and legal support (Figure 5.1) (World Health Organization, 2004).

Often multiple providers or programs offer different separate components of HIV/AIDS care and treatment services, although some programs offer comprehensive services within one site. Partnerships and collaboration, including a well-functioning referral system, among the various providers are therefore essential to enable timely access to appropriate services (Osborne, van Praag, and Jackson, 1997). Complicating the situation

Figure 5.1. Elements of Comprehensive Care

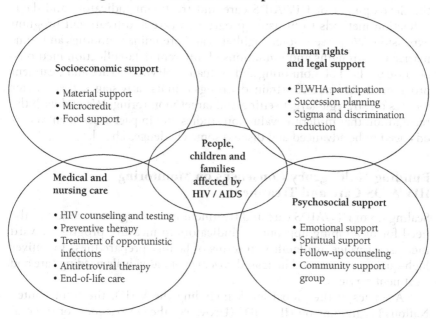

PLWHA: people living with HIV/AIDS.

is the need to address issues that fuel the HIV/AIDS epidemic and affect individuals' ability and willingness to access needed services: stigma, discrimination, fear, neglect, and impoverishment. Overall, HIV/AIDS care and treatment programs aim to

- Ensure equitable access to services
- Reduce HIV/AIDS-related morbidity and mortality
- Promote opportunities to prevent HIV transmission
- Improve the quality of life of people living with HIV/AIDS (World Health Organization, 2004)

Just as program planners and policymakers are deciding on the best approaches for scaling up HIV/AIDS care and treatment services, the monitoring and evaluation (M&E) community has begun to develop the necessary organizing frameworks, to prioritize key M&E questions, to implement appropriate data collection and analysis methods, and to focus on data use to enable learning and improve program implementation and success. The heightened attention and tremendous increased funding for HIV/AIDS care and treatment also comes with strong demands for accountability—the money must be tied to results.

In this chapter, we describe and critique our experience to date with the development of HIV/AIDS care and treatment indicators and data-collection methods to measure progress in care and treatment program expansion. We present some highlights and preliminary findings and summarize the strengths and limitations of different data-collection methods. Because the field of monitoring and evaluating HIV/AIDS care and treatment programs in resource-constrained settings is in its early stages, this chapter focuses on strategic target setting and target monitoring. We end with the recognition that in-depth evaluation studies and impact assessment methods need to be advanced and discuss some challenges ahead.

Building Multiagency Consensus on Monitoring HIV/AIDS Care and Treatment

Scaling up of HIV/AIDS care and treatment brings urgent attention to the need for developing appropriate indicators to measure progress toward increased service availability in terms of facility preparedness to deliver high-quality services and increased coverage of individuals needing care and treatment services.

Agencies at the global level, including the WHO, the Joint United Nations Programme on HIV/AIDS (UNAIDS), the U.S. Agency for International Development (USAID), the U.S. Centers for Disease Control and Prevention (CDC), and the World Bank have made substantial efforts over the past five years to develop key indicators for monitoring progress in various programmatic areas of a national HIV/AIDS response (Joint United Nations Programme on HIV/AIDS, 2000; U.S. Agency for International Development, 2003; Centers for Disease Control and Prevention, 2003; also see Chapters Two, Three, and Six, this issue). Although these indicator guides included a limited number of indicators for HIV/AIDS care and treatment, it was acknowledged that further development was needed. In addition, limited field-testing of HIV/AIDS care and treatment indicators in Thailand and Brazil gave further evidence of the need to update these indicators and to strengthen the methods for data collection. WHO spearheaded the revision and expansion of existing indicators with an eye to address emerging HIV/AIDS care and treatment issues. A series of expert panels and working group meetings was conducted from 2001 to 2003, involving technical experts, service planners, and service providers from a range of agencies and countries, as well as representatives from WHO and UNAIDS. Using the resulting set of updated indicators and methods, the international HIV/AIDS Care and Support M&E Technical Working Group conducted pilot tests in Kenya, Ethiopia, the Dominican Republic, and Cambodia. Host-country partners and members of the technical working group (including experts from WHO, UNAIDS, the United Nations Children's Fund, USAID, the CDC, the U.S. Health Resources and Services Administration, Family Health International, Horizons, MEASURE Evaluation, and ORC [Opinion

Research Corporation] Macro) jointly conducted and analyzed indicator pilot tests (Wolf and others, 2002). Health facility and population-based surveys were tested, and the survey questions were validated through qualitative interviews and focus groups, including people living with HIV/AIDS, caretakers and family members, orphans, and health care providers.

The pilot tests found that effective M&E of activities requires that health facilities routinely collect data and update records on HIV/AIDS care and support services. In some settings, the quantitative and qualitative nature of record keeping varies dramatically by facility. For example, morbidity and mortality data may be routinely compiled, but data on confirmed cases of HIV infection or AIDS may not be recorded. In addition, data on age and sex are often not available, limiting the inferences that can be drawn. Local adaptation of indicators is to be expected and encouraged to ensure relevance to national and subnational goals and objectives, but it is important to collect at least a subset of the standardized indicators to allow for cross-site and cross-country analysis. Overall, the pilot tests highlighted the importance of ensuring that the required resources and training are available so that M&E data can be routinely collected in a timely way. Other key challenges noted from the pilot tests are discussed in the section on data-collection approaches.

This joint indicator and methods improvement effort resulted in January 2004 in the publication of the *National AIDS Programs: A Guide to Monitoring and Evaluating HIV/AIDS Care and Support,* published and disseminated under the leadership of WHO (World Health Organization, 2004) (see Table 5.1 for illustrative indicators). The vision, then, is for donors, national governments, and international agencies to work together to support collection of these data. For WHO, the new care and treatment indicators provide the foundation for monitoring progress toward the "Treat 3 Million by 2005" goal. Using these essential indicators to provide the data needed for accountability requirements of numerous donor agencies is critical because parallel efforts and measures place unnecessary reporting burden on programs that receive multiple funding streams and must report to each donor in different ways.

By harmonizing indicators and methods as much as possible, staff have more time to spend delivering critical services rather than completing duplicative reports. Although extensive time and effort is required to establish the broad consensus between different stakeholders to develop and adopt these international standards, it seems worthwhile doing because it should lead to a more efficient system for tracking progress over time. WHO, the World Bank, the Global Fund, and the U.S. government have pledged to use international M&E norms and standards rather than creating new ones. This was formalized at the recent International Monetary Fund-World Trade Organization meeting in Washington, D.C., in April 2004 where members committed to supporting one M&E system at the national level (Joint United Nations Programme on HIV/AIDS, 2004).

Table 5.1. Illustrative Care, Support, and Treatment Indicators by Data Source

Indicator	Data Source or Methodol
Percentage of districts with at least one health facility providing antiretroviral combination herapy	Program reports, HMIS, or health facility survey
Percentage of people with advanced HIV infection receiving antiretroviral therapy	Program reports or HMIS plus modeling
Percentage of health care facilities that have the capacity and conditions to provide advanced-level HIV/AIDS care and support services, including antiretroviral therapy	Health facility survey
Percentage of health facilities with record-keeping systems for monitoring HIV/AIDS care and support	Health facility survey
Percentaqe of adults aged 18 to 59 who have been chronically ill for 3 or more months during the past 12 months whose households received basic external support in caring for the person	Population-based survey
Percentage of orphans and vulnerable children younger than 18 living in households that received basic external support in caring for the child	Population-based survey

HMIS, health management information system.
Source: World Health Organization, 2004.

Developing Best Practices in Data Collection

Care and treatment indicators are intended to provide information for local, national, and international programs on progress in the delivery of key HIV/AIDS services. M&E activities allow country health authorities and their partners to assess the extent to which programs are being implemented and are achieving the intended objectives. The information required to measure progress and success can be drawn from national surveys of HIV/AIDS care and treatment programs, from program reports or other documentation at the community or facility level, and from special studies. Building systems that effectively and accurately pull together the facility- and community-based program reporting is critical in understanding the national response from a comprehensive perspective. For this information to be easily accessible and used at the national level, it requires a central data warehouse or data system. Creating this central system is a highly challenging prospect but is likely to benefit health care beyond HIV/AIDS and serve as a model for M&E collaboration.

Monitoring data, which can be aggregated across sites and over time, can serve to highlight program components that may need to be strengthened or modified to reach specific goals. The two broad types of monitoring data required are program output indicators that are the direct result of

Table 5.2. Program-Level Care, Support, and Treatment Indicators

Program or Service Area	Number of Service Outlets/Programs	Number of Clients Served (by Gender)	Number of People Trained
Counseling and testing	X	X	X
Antiretroviral therapy	X	X	X
Basic clinical care and support for PLWHA	X	X	X
Tuberculosis care for PLWHA	X	X	X
Community care for PLWHA	X	X	X
Care for orphans and vulnerable children	X	X	X

PLWHA, people living with HIV/AIDS.

program activities and national outcome and impact indicators that measure the collective effect of all program partners in making progress toward national objectives. In this section, we present an overview of existing methods and systems and discuss the experience gained with pilot testing new survey instruments and methods. We compare the strengths and limitations of each of these data-collection methods.

Program output monitoring is commonly focused on the counts of persons receiving services (such as the number of people receiving HIV counseling and testing). Table 5.2 gives an example of the types of program-level data that are being collected for HIV/AIDS care, support, and treatment programs.

To capture program outputs, we rely largely on data reported from facility-based health management information systems (HMIS) and from routine program reports of community-based organizations and nongovernmental organization programs.

Facility-Based Health Management Information Systems. HMIS support the routine monitoring of many clinical services that take place, from HIV diagnosis through clinical monitoring and treatment. An example of routine facility-based HMIS information from counseling and testing services in Botswana is shown in Figure 5.2. The graph illustrates the increasing number of persons provided with HIV counseling and testing services within a network of sites in Botswana between 2000 and 2003.

The management function of HMIS extends to control of pharmaceuticals and related equipment and commodities. Tight control of antiretroviral drugs and opiates is an absolute necessity in the avoidance of black market sales and drug resistance. Primary data collection should be integrated at the facility level. These data will branch out into separate specialized data systems at higher levels, which then support standardized indicator reporting, commodities management, and other program functions at the national and international levels.

Building capacity in this area is a resource-intensive venture but one that provides benefits at every level—patient management, facility management,

Figure 5.2. Monthly Reports of HIV Counseling and Testing, April 2000–March 2003

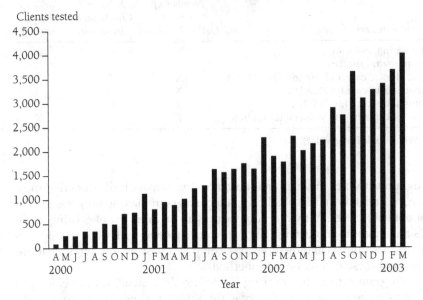

Source: Data compiled from the BOTUSA Project, a collaboration of the Botswana government and the U.S. Centers for Disease Control and Prevention.

national AIDS program management, and international program management. To build systems for quality data to be shared between different levels, HMIS need: the development of prototypes or strengthening of existing systems (including paper-based and computer systems and software) for semiannual reports; work with clinical centers and facilities to implement the HMIS, data quality control activities, and incentives; and the generation of reports, analysis, dissemination, and use of the data to improve programs.

Scaling up an HMIS requires considerable investment of time and resources, but it is critical for mainstreaming monitoring of care and treatment services. HMIS strengthening must take into account the following:

- Harmonize data elements, definitions, and training across different donor agencies
- Build on existing systems
- Integrate new technology where appropriate (for example, clinical monitoring software, smart cards)
- Build contractual obligations and incentives into programs for data collection and use
- Ensure that relevant data can be shared with stakeholders

- Facilitate two-way communication between providers and central program managers
- Assess data periodically for quality

The benefits of a standardized HMIS are clear; the downside is that providers in developing countries are often overworked, underpaid, and have low motivation to keep records. For an HMIS to be effective, it must be relatively simple to use and must provide obvious and quick benefits at the facility or provider level. It is important to remember that these systems not only will document HIV/AIDS but also will be useful for tracking tuberculosis, malaria, and child health. These multiple purposes may bring greater country ownership in the development and use of the data.

Community-Based Organization Program Reports. With the notable exception of the strong clinical care programs in Thailand and Brazil and a few demonstration projects scattered in different settings, community-based organizations historically provide most of the care and support in developing countries. These programs often rely on limited clinical staff and on teams of trained community health workers, often volunteers. They provide nursing care and emotional, psychosocial, and material support to the chronically ill and dying, the children and families of people living with HIV/AIDS, and AIDS orphans. Dedicated human resources to collect and manage information are understandably not often a high priority, and data quality is highly variable.

The success of antiretroviral therapy programs in health centers and hospitals depends on the effective interconnection with these community-based support and ancillary care programs and services, not only to provide additional needed services but also to aid with drug adherence and retention. In addition, because antiretroviral therapy is not a cure for AIDS, it will eventually fail and people become chronically ill, requiring community-based care services. The number of clients reached and the number of trained service providers outside of the facility setting, for example, are key pieces of information that should be analyzed in conjunction with the facility-based HMIS data to monitor access to life-prolonging services and continuity of care.

But unless these programs have ties to funding or other incentives, they will have low motivation for data collection. Educating community workers about the benefits that may be achieved by collecting information, including more efficient client management and advocacy for additional resources, is a necessary step. Tailored training and technical assistance on M&E is similarly important.

Population-Based Surveys. For the past three decades, national population household surveys have been a mainstay of reproductive and maternal-child health programs M&E. Many of the national outcome and impact HIV/AIDS indicators are derived from these surveys. The advantage of a

Table 5.3. External Support for Chronically Ill Persons (n = 92) in the Last Year and the Last Month

Type of Support for Chronically Ill Persons	Support in Last Year		Support in Last Month	
	No. (freq.)	%	No. (freq.)	%
Medical care	60	65	44	47
Medicines and medical supplies	35	38	26	32
Formal counseling	50	54	28	30
Emotional or spiritual support	32	35	30	33
Clothing	3	3	0	0
Extra food	11	12	7	8
Financial support	2	2	1	1
Help with household work	0	0	0	0
Training for caregiver	14	15	6	7
Legal services	0	0	0	0

Source: "Care and Support Pilot Test in Three Sites, Dominican Republic," 2003.

population-based survey is that information is collected directly from a representative sample of the general population, rather than only users of one or another program. As such, these surveys, if well designed and implemented, provide less biased estimates of knowledge, attitudes, practices, and program participation of the population. In addition to the vital information needed for prevention programs (such as risk behaviors), inclusion of care and treatment questions has significantly advanced the potential use of the survey data for program planning. These surveys also provide coverage information of relevant services, as illustrated in Table 5.3.

The information on key domains of care and support for chronically ill persons was obtained from the above-discussed pilot tests conducted in conjunction with the development of the WHO guide, *National AIDS Programmes: A Guide to Monitoring and Evaluating HIV/AIDS Care and Support* (World Health Organization, 2004). Table 5.3 shows reports from a pilot test in the Dominican Republic of various types of external medical and psychosocial support (beyond family friends and neighbors) chronically ill persons received within the last year and within the last month. Notable is that medical care, the most frequently cited type of support in three high-prevalence areas, was provided to only about two-thirds of those sampled within the last year and less than half in the last month. These types of data provide program managers with an assessment of the current situation on coverage of different types of comprehensive care and support services.

AIDS-specific surveys are relatively expensive and, therefore, should be done nationally on a periodic basis, about every two to three years depending on the level of the epidemic and available resources. Larger samples that allow regional or even district-level estimates are proportionately more costly. The larger demographic and health surveys are significantly more expensive and use larger sample sizes still, but these cover multiple health issues beyond HIV/AIDS and, therefore, are more cost-effective than AIDS-specific surveys. However, it is critical that the questions and methods of sampling are standardized between different surveys to compare findings over time. Donors can pool resources and work together to ensure that data are not just collected but used effectively to influence policy and improve programs.

The indicators that have been designed to track care and treatment of HIV/AIDS through national population surveys were designed with high-prevalence settings in mind. Therefore, a general population survey may not be the most cost-effective strategy for capturing care and treatment coverage within a concentrated epidemic context (that is, where only 1 to 2 percent of the general population is HIV-infected). In concentrated epidemics, such as in many countries in Asia and the Caribbean, the epidemic is largely focused in subpopulations, such as sex workers, injection-drug users, migrant laborers, or men who have sex with men. In these settings, tracking services in the general population is not efficient or effective when these services are targeting those most at risk. A general population survey in a low-prevalence setting means that it would take large sample sizes to find enough people who might be receiving care and treatment services. Many of the chronically ill and those who have died will not be related to AIDS, thus affecting the specificity of coverage estimates. Here, pilot testing demonstrated that adapting the national survey tool to a targeted sample drawn from networks of people living with AIDS, health facilities, and home-based care programs holds promise. The strength of this sampling method is that it is an invaluable tool in assessing care and treatment services for program planning purposes and for evaluating program service delivery over time. However, the sampling will not yield a representative (unbiased) national estimate.

Facility Surveys. Facility surveys complement population surveys and HMIS. Where population surveys can highlight coverage of services among the population, facility surveys can show capacity and quality (such as minimum standards) of clinical centers for the provision of basic and advanced HIV/AIDS care and treatment. The surveys give a snapshot of service availability and the quality of the national health care delivery system. Health facility surveys allow program planning and improvement related to the existence and availability of services, trained staff, drugs, equipment, guidelines and protocols, conditions, and capacity to monitor these services at the facility level. Basic methods for sampling and studying health facilities have been developed, and periodic health facility surveys, every two to three years, are recommended. These surveys also allow the collection of service utilization data when HMIS systems are weak but where facility record-keeping systems exist.

The facility-based indicators and instruments were developed and refined through pilot testing. They focus on basic-level HIV/AIDS services

Table 5.4. Basic-Level Facility-Capacity Indicators for HIV/AIDS Care and Support Services

Basic level HIV/AIDS Care and Support Services	Availability of the Indicated Item in the Service Delivery Area or the Facility if Proximity Is Not Relevant
System for testing and providing test results for HIV	Informed consent document, HIV test, records of test results, and clients receiving results
System and qualified staff for pre- and post-test counseling for HIV	Routine pre- and post-test counseling with trained provider, protocols to counseling, records of counseling, and counseling setting allows for visual and auditory privacy
Resources and supplies for providing specific health services relevant to HIV/AIDS	Service records, protocols for treatment, a trained provider, and the essential medications for tuberculosis, malaria, and sexually transmitted infections
Elements for preventing nosocomial infections	Soap and running water, a sharps box, chlorine decontaminating solution (if relevant), and clean latex gloves in each relevant service area
Trained staff and resources for providing basic interventions for treatment of PLWHA	Confidentiality protocols, treatment protocols, trained provider, and relevant medicines for opportunistic infections and palliative care, service records, and individual client charts or records
Preventive interventions for tuberculosis and pneumonia	Protocols and relevant medicine for prevention of tuberculosis and other opportunistic infections (such as pneumonia)

PLWHA, people living with HIV/AIDS.

(for example, services that could reasonably be provided from a health center) and advanced-level services. Advanced HIV/AIDS care services require a higher level of infrastructure, laboratory services, and trained service providers than those commonly found at health centers. Domains for these health facility-capacity indicators on basic HIV/AIDS care and treatment, as an example, are shown in Table 5.4.

For each level of HIV/AIDS care, specific services were identified and, within each service, specific items important for providing quality services and for monitoring minimum standards for service delivery. Services assessed by an inventory or checklist approach include counseling and testing for HIV, curative care and palliative care for people living with HIV/AIDS, services relevant to HIV/AIDS, and preventive interventions. Common elements assessed for each service are relevant policy documents (such as informed consent and confidentiality), treatment protocols, trained and supervised service providers, medicines, documentation for the services, and service settings that provide an adequate level of privacy. Figure 5.3 displays components for basic HIV/AIDS care within the facilities selected for the HIV/AIDS care and treatment indicators pilot test in Cambodia. Facility capacity scale up can be tracked over time in different geographical areas as well as nationally.

Figure 5.3. Cambodia Facility Survey Results, Showing Number of Facilities (*n* = 8) Having Each Component and All Components for Basic-Level Treatment and Preventive Interventions (8 of 13 Provide OI Treatment)

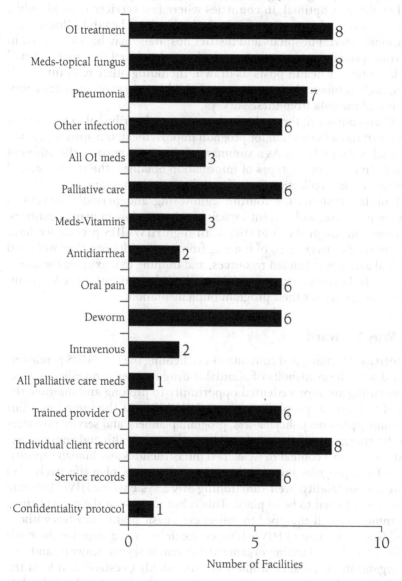

OI: opportunistic infections.

Source: Pretest data, outpatient units.

The potential benefits of institutionalizing routine periodic health facility surveys are promising. The challenge is that the surveys require highly trained clinical staff to conduct the interviews and are therefore expensive and timely. Sampling strategies are still being developed. Whereas a census of all facilities is optimal, in countries where few services exist in only a handful of hospitals, samples of only the higher-level health facilities, such as national referral hospitals and district hospitals, may be inventoried in full while a small random sample of the lower-level facilities, such as small health centers or health posts, is drawn. Including other relevant health issues, such as tuberculosis, malaria, and child health, may maximize countries' use of the data from these surveys.

When combined, the multiple data sources described above provide a system that has a foundation for program improvement, transparency, advocacy, and accountability. As a summary, Table 5.5 compares the different methods in terms of the types of information obtained, the recommended frequency of data collection, cost, feasibility, and limitations.

Building systems for routine monitoring and periodic surveys is resource intensive, and current capacity to do so is low in many countries. Therefore, although the countries with high HIV/AIDS prevalence have begun to receive large sums of funding from various donors, they will need technical assistance, human resources, and training to maximize the use of these funds. Less-resourced countries will need to prioritize the key components necessary for their program implementation.

The Way Forward

The increased funding and commitment to fighting the HIV/AIDS pandemic, coupled with the availability of affordable drug regimens and effective care, are providing an unprecedented opportunity to prolong and improve the lives of millions of people living with HIV/AIDS. At the same time, this opportunity presents policymakers, program planners, and service providers with the enormous challenge of rapidly scaling up health and community-based services in a context of weakened infrastructures and human capacity.

To track progress, improve programs and services, plan effectively, and ensure accountability, well-functioning M&E systems for HIV/AIDS care and treatment need to be in place. This is not the case at the present time. Governments are ill equipped to collect even basic health statistics without the additional burden of HIV/AIDS service delivery. To improve the environment for M&E, funding organizations, national governments, and service organizations must coordinate efforts quickly to establish at least the basic M&E tools and minimum human capacity to collect and use the data gathered effectively.

Global, national, and local levels need different data. Whereas international standards recommend that countries report on a small set of key national indicators for global tracking and cross-country comparisons, it is

Table 5.5. Comparison of Data-Collection Methods to Measure HIV/AIDS Care and Treatment Indicators

Method	Information Type Yielded	Frequency of Data Collection	Relative Cost	Feasibility	Limitations
Facility-based health management information system (HMIS)	Services delivered (facility-based)	Routine (semiannual reports)	Varies (high in most low-resource settings)	Medium	Facility-level human resource capacity for data collection and use is limited
Community-based program reports	Services delivered (home-based and community care programs)	Routine (semiannual reports)	Low	High	Data quality a major concern; poor standardization
Health facility survey	Health facility capacity (service availability)	Baseline and every 2 to 3 years	Medium to high	Medium to high	Limited to services provided out of health facilities
Population-based survey	Use of services provided at community level	Baseline and every 2 to 3 years	Medium to high	Designed for high-prevalence settings	Subject to reporting biases (disclosure, stigma); targeted samples needed for concentrated epidemic
Targeted evaluation studies	Various: intervention efficacy information, specific research questions and outcomes	Periodic, as needed	High	Medium	Costly (cohort studies); limited generalizability of studies

vital for national programs to have more information for management purposes. For instance, national program managers need data from different geographical areas within their country to plan for and monitor improvements in service coverage and capacity. They need to ensure equitable access to services by those in need. At the program level, even more detailed information is needed on the full range of services to ensure quality of services and to enable day-to-day management. For instance, although programs may be reporting only up to the national level the total number receiving HIV test results over a given period, for program improvement purposes they will want to know how many people refused HIV testing, where they were referred from, and whether they are indeed taking up the services (such as tuberculosis screening) to which they are referred. These different data needs are to be accommodated within a comprehensive M&E system with priority given to data needed at the national and subnational levels. As also discussed in Chapters Four and Six in this issue, the further harmonization of donor requirements is an issue for immediate attention by the existing global partnerships in M&E. Ensuring that data collection at the local level includes indicators that can feed up to the national level requires active participation of local governmental and nongovernmental organizations in the selection of key national indicators. Although a challenging process, Anie and Larbi (Chapter Eight, this issue) provide a good example of how to involve stakeholders at all levels in national M&E efforts.

Building capacity for M&E is vital to ensuring the success of the national response to HIV/AIDS. This requires considerable planning and long-term investment by donors and national program planners and may not be underestimated. To coordinate and use the data sources and methods discussed above, it is critical to assess and strengthen national and subnational M&E capacity and resources. Only by building adequate M&E capacity and a supportive culture for M&E will we ensure that data are meaningful, relevant, and used to improve programs.

To serve all data needs, a range of data-collection methods is required. However, these represent a considerable effort and cost and, therefore, need to be considered within a national strategic M&E plan that focuses on a phased implementation of M&E methods. The first responsibility is to ensure adequate monitoring. Programs can now take advantage of the newly developed care and treatment indicators and tried and tested methods, such as facility and household surveys, to gauge progress and current needs and trends in caring for people living with HIV/AIDS. Although management information systems at health care sites need considerable investment, both in the context of general health and targeted patient management in HIV/AIDS care and treatment, there is no real alternative to measuring coverage of vital services. A coordinated effort among global partners (UNAIDS; the World Bank; the Global Fund to Fight AIDS, Tuberculosis, and Malaria; WHO; and the U.S. government) to assess what can best be done to improve these systems is currently under way.

HIV care and treatment for developing countries is an evolving field, and the indicators and data-collection methods need to be revised periodically to ensure that they remain relevant and keep pace with the rapidly changing landscape of HIV/AIDS care and treatment services delivered in low-resource settings. Whereas tracking clinical services and capacity building for care and support are vital, other aspects are equally important. Specific indicators for the quality of care, quality of training, and human capacity development for providers, palliative care and stigma and human rights issues need to be developed. Studies are being carried out now and planned in the near future that will address these aspects of care and treatment not yet adequately covered.

Most indicators, however, are not designed to explain why a situation has or has not changed but to simply measure trends over time. In addition to data from routine HMIS, program reports, and population-based and facility surveys, additional special studies need to be conducted to address programmatic questions and determine successful models of care in different settings. A well-functioning patient management system provides a good platform for the collection and use of more in-depth data for program evaluation and research. Examples are studying survival rates, rates of opportunistic infections in clinic cohorts, and quality-of-life measures in relation to treatment models, such as using enhanced training with community outreach versus standard facility-based approaches. The evolving nature of HIV/AIDS care and treatment requires in-depth studies on the optimal delivery of services—for example, studies of antiretroviral combination therapy and adherence, the quality of care, training of health care providers, and the evolution of programs and methods for reducing stigma and discrimination within the health care system (World Health Organization, 2004). The main objective of such studies is to provide managers, administrators, and policymakers with the information they need to improve day-to-day activities or operations of HIV/AIDS prevention, care, and treatment programs.

Other special studies may be used to assess national program objectives. For example, document reviews of care, support, and treatment policies may compare the existence and content of national policies, strategies, and guidelines over time and the extent to which these include protection of the rights of people living with HIV/AIDS. Similarly, human capacity to deliver care and treatment has been identified as perhaps the most important barrier to implementation of care, support, and treatment services in low-resource settings. Special studies may review training curriculum and document the number of trained health professionals over time who serve in positions that they are trained for and key incentives and strategies for overcoming obstacles in this area. Qualitative data-collection techniques complement and enhance the interpretation and meaning of the data collected from the other methods listed here. It is from the actual voices and stories from providers and especially from people living with HIV/AIDS themselves that we learn how AIDS care and treatment affects their lives and the challenges to accessing services and factors that affect adherence to treatment regimens.

Care and treatment focuses on reducing morbidity and mortality and improving quality of life among people living with HIV/AIDS and their families. In most low-resource settings, population-based data on adult mortality generally and AIDS-related mortality in particular are scant. The ability to show an improved survival picture for countries experiencing an unprecedented treatment program expansion is crucial to advocacy efforts and a sustained programmatic response. Brazil's mortality surveillance system is a strong example here. Although vital registration and death certification systems are not yet well developed in most high-prevalence countries in Africa, some sentinel sites in key districts (such as in Tanzania) have developed sample vital registration systems that use verbal autopsy methods, allowing improved tracking of the cause and rates of disease-specific mortality. Developing these and related types of alternative, cost-effective approaches is critical to understanding the effects of HIV/AIDS treatment but also brings benefits to the broader health care delivery system beyond HIV/AIDS (World Health Organization, 2003b).

In conclusion, national governments in collaboration with international agencies have a full and comprehensive agenda for establishing sound M&E systems to guide effective HIV/AIDS care and treatment management, and a concerted effort is under way to implement this agenda. As we move forward, the main challenge is to actively involve stakeholders at different levels, including people living with HIV/AIDS, to ensure that the data collected serve their needs. If we fail to do this, the data quality and sustainability of data-collection efforts are in question, leading potentially to an enormous opportunity cost of human and financial resources dedicated to data that are inadequately used.

References

Centers for Disease Control and Prevention. *Monitoring the Global AIDS [Acquired Immunodeficiency Syndrome] Program: Indicator Guide for Annual Reporting.* Atlanta: Centers for Disease Control and Prevention, 2003.

De Lay, P., Ernberg, G., and Stanecki, K. "Introduction." In P. Lamptey and H. Gayle (eds.), *HIV/AIDS Prevention and Care in Resource-Constrained Settings: A Handbook for the Design and Management of Programs.* Arlington, Va.: Family Health International, 2001.

Joint United Nations Programme on HIV/AIDS. *National AIDS Programmes: A Guide to Monitoring and Evaluation.* Geneva: Joint United Nations Programme on HIV/AIDS, 2000.

Joint United Nations Programme on HIV/AIDS. *Monitoring the Declaration of Commitment on HIV/AIDS Guidelines on the Construction of Core Indicators.* Geneva: Joint United Nations Programme on HIV/AIDS, 2002.

Joint United Nations Programme on HIV/AIDS. "Landmark Agreement Reached in Fight Against AIDS." Press release. Washington, D.C.: Joint United Nations Programme on HIV/AIDS, 2004.

Osborne, C., van Praag, E., and Jackson, H. "Models of Care for Patients With HIV/AIDS." *AIDS*, 1997, *11*(Suppl. B), S135–S141.

U.S. Agency for International Development. *Expanded Response Guide to Core Indicators for Monitoring and Reporting on HIV/AIDS Programs*. Washington, D.C.: U.S. Agency for International Development, 2003.

Wolf, R. C., and others. "Pilot Testing HIV/AIDS Care, Support and Treatment Indicators in High Prevalence Countries in Africa: Lessons Learned From the Care and Support Monitoring and Evaluation Working Group." In *Program and Abstracts of the 14th International AIDS Conference*. Barcelona: July 7–12, 2002. Abstract TuPpD2065.

World Health Organization *Treating 3 Million by 2005: Making It Happen—The WHO Strategy*. Geneva: World Health Organization, 2003a.

World Health Organization. *Improving Systems for Monitoring and Measurement of Vital Events: An Issues Paper Prepared for the Health Metrics Network*. Geneva: World Health Organization, 2003b.

World Health Organization. *National AIDS Programs: A Guide to Monitoring and Evaluating HIV/AIDS Care and Support*. Geneva: World Health Organization, 2004.

R. CAMERON WOLF *is the senior technical adviser for monitoring and evaluation at the Office of HIV/AIDS, U.S. Agency for International Development, Washington, D.C.*

GEORGE BICEGO *is the regional adviser for strategic information in Southern Africa, Global AIDS Program, U.S. Centers for Disease Control and Prevention.*

KATHERINE MARCONI *is director of strategic information and evaluation in the Office of the U.S. Global AIDS Coordinator, Washington, D.C.*

RUTH BESSINGER *is an epidemiologist and evaluation analyst at ORC Macro, Calverton, Maryland.*

ERIC VAN PRAAG *is the country director for Family Health International in Tanzania and is a public health expert in HIV care, treatment, and support.*

SHANTI NORIEGA-MINICHIELLO *is a technical officer in the Measurement and Health Information Systems Department of the World Health Organization, Geneva, Switzerland.*

GREGORY PAPPAS is the medical director of the Futures Group, Washington, D.C.

NANCY FRONCZAK is the Survey Provision Assessment survey coordinator through MEASURE DHS/ORC Macro, Calverton, Maryland.

GREET PEERSMAN is the technical deputy director of the Monitoring and Evaluation Team for the Global AIDS Program at the U.S. Centers for Disease Control and Prevention, Atlanta, Georgia.

RENÉE K. FIORENTINO is the monitoring and evaluation adviser to the National AIDS Commission of Rwanda through MEASURE Evaluation/John Snow, Inc.

DEBORAH RUGG is the associate director of the Monitoring and Evaluation Team for the Global AIDS Program at the U.S. Centers for Disease Control and Prevention, Atlanta, Georgia.

JOHN NOVAK is the monitoring and evaluation adviser to the U.S. Agency for International Development, Washington, D.C.

6

An operational plan for monitoring and evaluation with a detailed budget is an essential step in moving from an indicator set to a functioning monitoring and evaluation system. Experience suggests that this will happen only with appropriate funding incentives.

World Bank Contribution to Building National HIV/AIDS Monitoring and Evaluation Capacity in Africa: Going Beyond Indicator Development and Conceptual Training

David Wilson

International commitment to the human immunodeficiency virus-acquired immunodeficiency syndrome (HIV/AIDS) epidemic has grown rapidly in recent years, stimulated by the leadership of the Joint United Nations Programme on HIV/AIDS (UNAIDS) and its cosponsors and supported by a range of new mechanisms. These include the World Bank's Multi-Country AIDS Program (World Bank, 1999), the Global Fund to Fight AIDS, Tuberculosis and Malaria (Global Fund) (2003), and most recently, the U.S. President's Emergency Plan for AIDS Relief (Office of the U.S. Global HIV/AIDS Coordinator, 2003). Global HIV/AIDS spending grew from an estimated US$300 million in 1996 to US$2.8 billion in 2002 (World Bank, 2003a). The critical need to ensure that available resources are used effectively places unprecedented responsibility on monitoring and evaluation (M&E). Improving M&E, in turn, requires a sustained commitment to capacity building and systems development, particularly in countries confronted by limited public sector capacity and human resources, problems exacerbated by widespread poverty and AIDS mortality.

In this chapter, I summarize the World Bank's recent experiences with M&E capacity-building approaches in support of the development of national M&E frameworks and operational M&E plans and budgets, primarily within the context of the World Bank's Multi-Country AIDS

NEW DIRECTIONS FOR EVALUATION, no. 103, Fall 2004 © Wiley Periodicals, Inc.

Program. This program was initiated in 2000 as a long-term commitment of at least fifteen years to prevent HIV/AIDS and mitigate its impact in Africa (World Bank, 1999). By 2003, US$1 billion had been approved for twenty-four established and eight pending country and subregional projects in Africa (World Bank, 2004a). Through its multicountry AIDS program, the World Bank has joined UNAIDS and other United Nations and bilateral agencies as major partners of national AIDS councils in Africa. These multisectoral, national coordinating bodies are typically the World Bank's point of entry and its primary focus for M&E capacity-building support.

To strengthen its own institutional capacity to support HIV/AIDS programs around the world, the World Bank established the Global HIV/AIDS Program in 2002 with UNAIDS support and, within that, an M&E unit. The M&E team's overarching objective is to strengthen national M&E capacity and M&E systems through sustainable approaches. Capacity-building initiatives reflect increased financial resources, human resource development, focused training, and intensive technical assistance. Interactions with thirty-one national and subregional AIDS authorities in the course of eighty-five support visits in the past three years have led to several major lessons learned (World Bank, 2003b, 2004a). These form the content of this chapter.

Building Comprehensive M&E Systems

Generally, international M&E efforts have devoted much time to indicators at the expense of the M&E systems required to collect indicator data (World Bank, 2003b). Worse still, these efforts have unwittingly given country partners the erroneous impression that a comprehensive list of indicators constitutes an M&E plan. Most countries have an M&E strategy and have drafted indicators. However, far fewer countries have progressed to a detailed, typically five-year operational plan that specifies precisely when, how, and by whom each M&E product is collected and how data flow from tier to tier, together with a detailed M&E budget that fully reflects the recurrent and incremental costs of each M&E product.

The World Bank AIDS program's guiding principle is to promote one, comprehensive, national M&E system (Joint United Nations Programme on HIV/AIDS, 2001) that has the following components:

- *One national M&E information system,* including a flowchart that specifies precisely how data from each M&E component and each level are collated into the single overall national repository, ideally a Web-accessible database.
- *Biological surveillance and behavioral surveillance:* conducting regular, credible, and affordable HIV and behavioral surveillance among both general population groups and priority population groups, in keeping with international best practice
- *Essential research:* identifying priority research questions and effectively supporting credible research in HIV/AIDS prevention and care

- *Program activity monitoring:* tracking HIV/AIDS-related activities and services through a monitoring system that ensures that all partners submit regular, structured program reports that are externally verified
- *Financial monitoring:* tracking expenses and cost services and corroborating program activity reports

Coordination and Implementation of a Comprehensive M&E System

National AIDS councils were established under the leadership of UNAIDS as high-level coordination and advocacy bodies (Joint United Nations Programme on HIV/AIDS, 2003). Through the World Bank AIDS Program, the Global Fund, and bilateral donors, national AIDS councils have become grant-making bodies making subgrants to hundreds of community-based organizations. However, there are concerns that the demands of grant making have transformed national AIDS councils into banks, with limited time to absorb or manage technical data. In contrast, national AIDS programs within the ministries of health have a wealth of technical expertise but limited opportunities to inject this expertise into the national AIDS councils' decision making.

The World Bank strongly supports UNAIDS' view that national AIDS councils should be coordination, not implementation, bodies. National AIDS councils must find ways of reducing or delegating the administrative burden of grant making and must develop mechanisms to ensure a greater infusion of expertise from national AIDS programs. Table 6.1 provides an example of how national AIDS councils can devolve specific M&E responsibilities to specialist national institutions.

Table 6.1. Shared Responsibilities for Coordinating and Implementing a Comprehensive M&E System

M&E Component	Responsible Agencies
Overall national M&E architecture	NAC assisted by the ministry of health's NAP
Biological surveillance	Ministry of health's NAP assisted by the central statistical office for population-based HIV prevalence surveys and other ministry of health units for antenatal surveys
Behavioral surveillance	Ministry of health's NAP assisted by the behavioral surveillance committee and implemented by universities, research institutions, or research or consulting firms
Essential research	Ministry of health's NAP, universities, and research institutions
Program activity monitoring	Health sector: ministry of health's NAP Social sectors: accounting or consulting firm
Financial monitoring	Accounting firm

NAC, national AIDS councils; NAP, national AIDS program.

Implementing the Components of a Comprehensive M&E System

In consultation with global and country partners, the World Bank AIDS Program has formulated an operational definition with discrete data products and performance criteria for each M&E component of a comprehensive M&E system (see below) (World Bank, 2003a). The operational definition places great emphasis on the effective use of M&E products to improve decision making and programming:

Overall National M&E Information System
• Integrated national database and flowchart
• Annual M&E business plan demonstrating active and effective use of M&E data for program progress review and program modification

Biological Surveillance
• Annual antenatal surveillance using international protocols, with external review
• Five-yearly general population surveys using international protocols, with external review (in high-prevalence countries)
• Semiannual surveys using international protocols, with external review, of priority population groups, including sex workers and at least two other priority groups relevant to HIV transmission dynamics (such as injecting-drugs users, men having sex with men, uniformed services, or mobile populations)

Behavioral Surveillance
• Semiannual general population-based surveys using guidelines of demographic and health surveys or AIDS indicator surveys, with external review
• Semiannual surveys using behavioral surveillance surveys guidelines, with external review, of priority population groups, including sex workers and at least two other priority groups relevant to HIV transmission dynamics (such as injecting-drugs users, men having sex with men, uniformed services, or mobile populations)

Health Facility Surveillance
• Three- to five-yearly health facility surveys of coverage and quality of key HIV/AIDS services

Essential Research
• At least two intervention studies evaluating critical HIV/AIDS transmission dynamics, prevention, or both, and care and support interventions, in collaboration with academic and external experts
• Evidence of an effective strategy for dissemination and application of research findings

Program Activity Monitoring
• Semiannual community surveys (combined with the population-based and priority population behavioral surveys mentioned above) to assess the quantity, quality, and coverage of community HIV/AIDS services

- Program activity reporting, with independent validation, by national AIDS council grant recipients
- Program activity reporting, with independent validation, of all implementing partners supported by national AIDS councils and other agencies so that countries obtain a comprehensive summary of services provided
- Program analysis, including service delivery comparisons, and evidence that this program analysis is influencing grant-making and capacity-building strategies

Financial Monitoring

- Financial reporting, with independent auditing, of national AIDS council grant recipients
- Financial analysis, including unit-cost comparisons and, if possible, cost-effectiveness modeling, of different interventions, program models, and service providers and evidence that this financial analysis is influencing grant-making and capacity-building strategies

Supervision and Review

- Annual program review, based on M&E products of each of the above components, with evidence that the program review uses M&E data to make strategic program improvements

For example, Malawi developed a two-part M&E plan (National AIDS Commission, 2003). Part A is the conceptual framework, which includes the theoretical foundations of the system, the logical framework, and the indicators. Part B is the operational plan, which is intended to be a practical, self-contained "road map" for M&E implementation. It summarizes the indicators and provides a detailed operational definition of each indicator; includes a detailed implementation plan that spells out when, how, by whom, and at what cost each indicator will be collected; and presents data-flow diagrams for each indicator. The operational plan also includes a detailed budget and outlines a clear process to ensure that M&E data are actively used at each level to improve program management and performance. Although it took one year to develop the Malawi M&E plan, subsequent experience demonstrates that it provides a basis for rapid emulation elsewhere. Namibia and Swaziland, for example, developed similar plans in three months.

An operational plan with a detailed budget is an essential step in moving from an indicator set to a functioning M&E system. However, this will happen only if the funding culture creates genuine incentives to do so.

Incentives for Functioning M&E Systems

M&E is usually viewed as a technical discipline with little consideration of the wider management context. However, the World Bank AIDS program and the Global Fund provide an interesting comparison that underscores the centrality of incentives (World Bank, 2004a). Quite simply, organizations are likely to develop functioning M&E systems if there are incentives to do so.

The World Bank AIDS program recognizes the importance of M&E but does not require partners to have functioning M&E systems to receive AIDS funds. In contrast, the Global Fund, with its emphasis on results-based disbursement, requires partners to establish and maintain functioning M&E systems to receive disbursements (Global Fund, 2003). As a result, Global Fund recipients prioritize M&E. The most urgent requests for M&E technical assistance from the World Bank come from Global Fund partners, not from the World Bank's program partners. Moreover, whereas requests for World Bank M&E assistance come overwhelmingly from task managers within the World Bank, Global Fund–related requests for M&E assistance come directly from national recipients. Global Fund recipients develop M&E systems far more rapidly, prioritizing staff and resources to do so. Global Fund recipients willingly spend their own resources to develop M&E systems, including contracting international specialists, which the World Bank funding recipients are reluctant to do. Similarly, several countries have established M&E posts specifically for Global Fund projects. Although this may not contribute to the shared goal of one national M&E system, it does demonstrate urgency, purposefulness, and country ownership.

A similar comparison may be made with financial management. All World Bank program partners have established functioning financial management systems because these systems are required for further disbursements. In contrast, few functioning program management systems are in place because these are not linked to disbursements.

Expenditure analysis further demonstrates the low priority assigned to M&E in the absence of specific incentives. In the World Bank's AIDS program, M&E is typically subsumed under the coordination and capacity-building component (World Bank, 2003b). However, many countries quickly exhaust this category on general expenses, such as salaries, offices, transport, and equipment, leaving no funds to implement essential M&E activities. This affirms the importance of incentives for M&E and also highlights the need to establish a separate, nonfungible M&E budget.

The conclusion is clear: without credible incentives to establish functioning M&E systems, intensive M&E technical assistance and capacity-building support may be insufficient. In recognition of this, the interim review of the World Bank Multi-Country HIV/AIDS Program for Africa advocated either moving toward results-based disbursements or making the establishment of functioning M&E systems a prerequisite for future World Bank support.

Need for Management-Oriented M&E and Knowledge Management

Few M&E frameworks are designed as management tools (World Bank, 2004a). They tend to emphasize longer-term health benefits, such as safer sexual behavior at the outcome level or reduced prevalence of sexually transmitted infections including HIV at the impact level. Output targets, such as voluntary counseling and testing services to be expanded by 50 percent in three years, tend to be broad and long term. If M&E is to be useful to managers, it must be much more management oriented and designed to provide more immediate and continuous feedback on performance.

The Global Fund has confronted this issue earlier than other donor agencies. To implement a quarterly results-based disbursement system, recipients must establish what targets are realistic every three months. This leads to specific, relevant, implementation-oriented targets. In the case of a treatment program, for example, these may relate to the development of treatment guidelines, the preparation of a training course for clinicians, training of trainers, and the training of a designated number of clinicians. Subsequent targets need to reflect achievements and identify appropriate targets for the next quarter. Such an approach needs supplementary programmatic indicators, in addition to nationally defined outcome and impact indicators, to be specified in an agreed-on work plan.

Overall, national AIDS councils have had limited success in establishing functioning systems that monitor program activity (World Bank, 2004a). Several common pitfalls are evident in existing systems. First, some national AIDS councils limit program activity monitoring to general indicators, such as the percentage of districts with voluntary counseling and testing centers. Yet, this information is of limited value unless one knows how many people are using the voluntary counseling and testing centers. Second, some national AIDS councils collect primarily narrative program reports. They quickly receive more reports than they can work through (in some cases, several thousand), and the information contained is too heterogeneous to summarize across reports. Third, some national AIDS councils permit partners to report in their own format and on their own indicators. This means that indicators cannot be aggregated at the district, regional, or national level, resulting in an inability to report on the scale of core services delivered, such as the number of people living with HIV/AIDS receiving support and the number of AIDS patients receiving care. In this case, national AIDS councils may try to extract what data they can from individual reports, but the data represent a severe underestimate of actual services delivered. Fourth, some national AIDS councils have prepared standardized reports, but these reports are often too complex to be feasible. For example, one national AIDS council requests partners to report on peer education beneficiaries reached by age group and by target group.

In response to these specific challenges, the World Bank AIDS program has developed a simple, standardized, one-page reporting form covering thirteen priority HIV/AIDS prevention, care, support, and mitigation indicators (World Bank, 2004b). The World Bank encourages national AIDS councils to include this form in their partnership agreements and to require the completed form to be submitted together with financial reports to receive the next disbursement.

At least half of the World Bank AIDS grants are typically reserved for the civil society component. Under this component, national AIDS councils are funding a wide range of HIV/AIDS prevention, care, support, and mitigation initiatives. There may be scope to improve the quality of these initiatives through enhanced knowledge management (World Bank, 2004a). Knowledge management requires the identification and promotion of good practices, and effective monitoring of the scale and quality of initiatives supported to ensure they contain the essential elements of good practice. In the future, the World Bank proposes to assist with knowledge management by identifying good practices through rigorous evidence-based analysis; defining the critical elements of success and distilling these into simple, accessible guidelines; preparing checklists to assess whether the critical elements are present; and developing procedures to implement the checklists.

A Coordinated Multiagency Response to M&E Needs

Despite increased financial support for M&E from national and international development partners, funding is often short term and limited to a specific M&E activity, such as a behavioral survey (World Bank, 2003b). In addition, some donors can support M&E technical assistance but not operational expenses. National M&E plans are thus held hostage to funding vagaries, and national AIDS councils and national AIDS programs are required to prepare annual M&E "shopping lists," which may or may not be funded in full. It is vital to establish long-term M&E funding, including both operational funding and technical assistance support. Countries cannot establish functioning M&E systems or promote sound data analysis and data use without long-term M&E plans and committed resources. There is great opportunity for complementary support between donor agencies. Whereas the World Bank can easily fund long-term, in-country, operational costs, the U.S. government agencies have effective mechanisms to provide international technical assistance.

The World Bank is committed to coalesce and pool support with national and international partners behind a small number of high-quality data products, including national antenatal HIV surveillance, priority-group HIV surveillance, national household HIV/AIDS surveys, and large-scale health facility surveys. The underlying rationale is that the proliferation of small-scale biological and behavioral studies of indeterminate quality has clouded clear interpretation—in short, a bad survey is often worse than none at all.

Both biological and behavioral surveillance are relatively well developed. The World Health Organization (WHO), UNAIDS, the U.S. Centers for Disease Control and Prevention (CDC), and the U.S. Agency for International Development (USAID) ensure sound antenatal HIV surveillance in many countries (World Health Organization, 1999). Population-based HIV-prevalence surveys are being extended to a growing number of countries, including Mali, Zambia, and Kenya (MEASURE [Measure and Evaluation to Assess and Use Results project]/ORC [Opinion Research Corporation] Macro, 2003). General population-based behavioral surveys supported by USAID are increasingly widespread (World Health Organization, 1999). Behavioral surveys in priority population groups, using guidelines and tools developed by UNAIDS and Family Health International, have been done in several contexts (Family Health International, 2004), although there is scope for expansion.

However, there is far more support for biological and behavioral surveillance in eastern and southern Africa than in central or West Africa (World Bank, 2004a). This is primarily because the U.S. government, the largest provider of M&E technical assistance and resources through USAID and the CDC, works principally in eastern and southern Africa. Moreover, Cote d'Ivoire's civil war has vitiated Abidjan's historical role as a source of technical expertise for much of francophone Africa. Thus, the World Bank gratefully acknowledges international technical collaboration from the U.S. government agencies in eastern and southern Africa and tries to broker support from international agencies or regional centers of expertise to enhance surveillance in central and West Africa.

The picture is similar for research support (World Bank, 2004a). It is generally well developed in eastern and southern African countries, with substantial domestic research capacity and significant international research funding and partnerships, but far less developed in many central and West African countries. The World Bank encourages research in all countries receiving World Bank AIDS funding. In eastern and southern Africa, it helps to identify and promote effectiveness research in HIV/AIDS prevention and care. In central and West Africa, the World Bank is proactive in promoting research in general to address major knowledge gaps.

For a variety of reasons, program-activity monitoring is the greatest single challenge (World Bank, 2004c). First, health-related program-activity monitoring relies to a great extent on a functioning health information system, and despite significant technical assistance and funding, few countries have adequately functioning health information systems (see Chapter Five, this issue). Second, the major international funder of HIV/AIDS services, the U.S. government agencies, for the most part, channel resources through cooperating agencies, usually large international nongovernmental organizations who in turn form partnerships with local agencies. These cooperating agencies generally have excellent program-activity monitoring systems. For example, Population Services International has outstanding systems for tracking condom sales by country, geographical area, sales outlet, and time period. These data are used to make national and international comparisons, to set performance goals, to improve programming, and to enhance efficiencies. Similarly, Family Health International has well-developed systems to monitor the quantity and quality of voluntary counseling and testing services. Because the U.S. government agencies are therefore able to monitor the services they support through their cooperating agencies, they have historically had limited incentive to strengthen national program-activity monitoring systems. Third, support to national AIDS councils has generally not been linked to effective performance, which has reduced the incentives to develop simple and effective program-activity monitoring systems. Fourth, major international development partners have tended to conclude that it is too difficult to establish ongoing information-gathering systems and have turned to episodic surveys that, with adequate funding and international technical assistance, can be reliably executed.

The Multi-Country AIDS Program places the World Bank in a different position. It is providing resources to numerous national AIDS councils, who in turn are providing grants to hundreds of implementing partners. National AIDS councils, therefore, require simple, structured program-activity data that indicate what services grant recipients are providing and how well they are performing. Furthermore, these program-activity data must be externally verifiable. Thus, the national AIDS councils and the World Bank share an interest in the development of simple program-activity monitoring systems.

The World Bank has obvious strengths in financial monitoring, which dovetail with its interests in program-activity monitoring. Wherever possible, the World Bank recommends that program-activity and financial monitoring be combined and entrusted to a single entity. Ideally, the same agency will verify both program activity and financial data. Because the same operations and personnel may be used, combining financial and program monitoring makes them affordable and allows for data cross-verification. In addition, because financial monitoring is usually the most developed component of monitoring, it makes sense to link program monitoring to the strongest foundation.

In summary, in many eastern and southern African countries where there are several international development partners supporting surveillance and research, the World Bank focuses its support on integrating different data streams into one overall M&E system and on program-activity monitoring linked to financial monitoring (World Bank, 2004c). In many central and West African countries, where there are fewer development partners supporting M&E, the World Bank addresses the entire spectrum of M&E, sometimes supporting the first credible antenatal surveillance the country has undertaken and building upward from there. In all contexts, the World Bank encourages countries to use World Bank resources to fund M&E, particularly long-term operational costs, and plays a facilitation and brokerage role in linking countries to national, regional, and international sources of M&E technical support.

Beyond Conceptual Training to Practical Field Support

The World Bank AIDS program's analysis of M&E resources and needs led to one major conclusion: there are simply too few M&E personnel available at all levels. Many national AIDS council M&E units are inadequately or inappropriately staffed, and there are too few national M&E experts available to support the national AIDS councils. Similarly, there are too few international M&E specialists available to provide appropriate, field-based M&E support when needed and too few international M&E personnel to coordinate global M&E assistance.

The World Bank and other international agencies have generally underestimated the true extent of M&E capacity-building needs (World Bank, 2004a). For the first two years, World Bank M&E support was largely limited to one part-time position. Today, the World Bank has three full-time M&E staff to support the US$1 billion program portfolio. Although it is a funding mechanism, not a technical agency, the Global Fund has only two M&E staff to support a US$2 billion program portfolio. Within countries, national AIDS councils similarly underestimated the scale of the capacity-building and systems development needs confronting them. National AIDS councils typically appoint one or two M&E officers and are hesitant to contract national M&E specialists to design, document, test, and transfer functioning M&E systems.

Although there is increasing lexical and conceptual convergence in M&E philosophies and approaches at the global level, this convergence has not yet filtered to the country level, where conflicting definitions and conceptions of M&E vitiate coordinated progress. Many countries still have several indicator sets and data-collection systems tailored to different donors. An intensified effort is required to achieve harmonized understanding and approaches at the country level.

There is also an urgent need to complement conceptual training with more intensive field support, particularly responsive expert technical assistance at national and subnational levels. Without such assistance, the increased investment in M&E will not yield optimal returns. For example, there are several countries in central and West Africa who intend to undertake major biological, behavioral, and health facility surveys without adequate national capacity to ensure quality. So the establishment of an accessible global pool of resources and experts to provide expert technical assistance at short notice has been identified as an interagency priority.

As noted above, there are marked disparities in the distribution of financial and human resources available to support M&E in different geographical regions (World Bank, 2003b). Whereas many eastern and southern African countries with high HIV prevalence enjoy adequate and in some cases excessive amounts of M&E funding and technical assistance, other countries have extremely limited national capacity and little or no access to M&E funding or technical assistance. Some high-prevalence countries have more M&E technical assistance than they can absorb or coordinate, leading to illogical fragmentation. For example, in two such countries, one group of M&E consultants worked with national AIDS council members on the development of a logical framework, and other M&E consultants worked concurrently but entirely separately with other national AIDS council members on national indicators. Several countries in this region have more than one national M&E plan, developed with assistance from different M&E partners.

In contrast, many countries in central and West Africa, such as Sierra Leone, Niger, or Guinea Bissau, have almost no access to vitally needed M&E technical assistance. Similarly, countries in the Horn of Africa, especially those experiencing or emerging from conflict, have little access to M&E funding or technical assistance. Small but high-prevalence countries in southern Africa, such as Swaziland and Lesotho, also receive limited support. The rapid M&E response pool, advocated for above, should have funds that are not earmarked to specific countries to enable a focus on the most underserved countries.

The enormity of this challenge should not obscure the fact that there have been demonstrable, sustained improvements in M&E capacity at the international and national levels. Internationally, major development partners have strengthened their M&E units through increasing their staff and M&E budgets. In addition, the U.S. government agencies are recruiting a field corps of M&E professionals (see Chapter Four, this issue), and UNAIDS has appointed an M&E director and is also recruiting M&E professionals for in-country residential M&E support. M&E guidelines have been prepared for national AIDS councils and national AIDS programs and for major intervention areas including youth, voluntary counseling and testing, prevention of mother-to-child transmission, HIV/AIDS care and treatment, and orphans and vulnerable children (see Chapter Five, this issue). Increased funding for M&E is being provided through a variety of agencies. USAID, the CDC, UNAIDS, and MEASURE/University of North Carolina have established ongoing M&E training courses in Africa and Asia, which have increased M&E conceptual understanding (MEASURE/University of North Carolina, 2002). Nationally, M&E units have been established in many national AIDS councils and national AIDS programs. Antenatal HIV surveillance has been strengthened, population-based HIV and behavioral surveillance is being expanded, and health facility surveys are being introduced to monitor HIV-related services.

The World Bank's contribution has focused on the establishment of a global M&E team with three full-time staff, an international country support team of consultant M&E specialists, and a nucleus of national M&E experts to assist their national AIDS councils. Through the country support team, the World Bank has also assisted national AIDS councils with the recruitment of appropriate M&E staff.

The country support team consists of M&E specialists who can be deployed to provide M&E support to thirty-eight countries, including World Bank AIDS funding recipients. The support is not limited to World Bank partnerships but also extends to UNAIDS, the Global Fund, and to countries directly. By 2003, ten international M&E specialists had been recruited, of whom seven are Africans. These M&E specialists were purposefully chosen to reflect a diversity of medical, epidemiological, social

Table 6.2. M&E-Related Field Visits of Country Support Teams

Country	Number of Visits	Country	Number of Visits
Benin	1	Kenya	7
Burkina Faso	2	Lagos-Abidjan Corridor	1
Cameroon	1	Madagascar	3
Cape Verde	5	Malawi	4
Congo-Brazzaville	2	Mauritania	1
Congo-DR	1	Mozambique	5
Djibouti	1	Namibia	2
Eritrea	3	Rwanda	2
Ethiopia	4	Senegal	4
Gambia	3	Sierra Leone	5
Ghana	1	Swaziland	10
Great Lakes	3	Tanzania	2
Guinea	2	Togo	1
Horn of Africa	2	Uganda	3
Lesotho	1	Zambia	1
		Zimbabwe	1

science, and evaluation experience, reflecting the World Bank's conviction that M&E is profoundly interdisciplinary. Most of the M&E specialists are based in Africa, where they can be deployed rapidly and economically to ensure the best use of World Bank M&E resources. Each M&E specialist supports an M&E portfolio of two to four countries and are selected on the basis of criteria such as relevant language skills, previous regional or country experience, ability to travel rapidly and economically from their residence to the country, and specific M&E skills relevant to country priorities. To date, the country support team has undertaken three training courses in Africa designed to ensure a harmonized approach between the consultant M&E specialists and to equip them with essential M&E skills.

By early 2004, the country support team had made eighty-five M&E field support visits to thirty-one countries or projects (see Table 6.2), providing about ten thousand person-hours of intensive M&E support. This focused on the following key steps in support of national M&E systems: assessment of M&E needs and priorities; development of a national M&E framework, including indicators; development of an M&E operational plan, including a detailed M&E budget; strengthening and integrating biological and behavioral surveillance; strengthening health facility surveys; enhancing research; strengthening program-activity and financial monitoring systems; M&E training for national AIDS councils and implementing partners; and case-specific M&E assistance (World Bank, 2004c). Another example of M&E support is the way that country support team members assisted in the development of protocols for pooled funding to the national AIDS council in Malawi. To date, four major development partners, including the World Bank, have agreed to pool their funds. They also assisted with the development of national M&E guidelines, including program-activity monitoring guidelines, that all development partners agreed to use instead of their own guidelines, whether they are pooling their funding or not (National AIDS Commission, 2003).

To promote sustainable approaches, country support team members try to identify and work with a national M&E expert, transferring necessary skills to the national M&E expert so that this expertise remains an accessible and sustainable source of support to national AIDS councils (World Bank, 2004c). Where possible, this in-country M&E expert is appointed as an advisor to the national AIDS council so that his or her primary affiliation and accountability is to the national AIDS council. Once a national in-country M&E expert is appointed, country support team members provide inception training and subsequently conduct regular support visits and e-mail and telephone contact.

The national in-country M&E experts are needed in addition to and complement the role of the M&E officers within national AIDS councils. Above all, national AIDS council M&E officers have an important representation and communication role within the councils, often preparing briefs for their directors or boards and deputizing for senior officials. Hence, they cannot protect adequate time to develop and document an entire M&E system. In addition, many national AIDS council M&E officers have skills in areas other than systems development and documentation. In contrast, the national M&E expert can be narrowly selected for the required skills.

Conclusion

With the experience of its global HIV/AIDS program, the World Bank has learned important lessons that are applicable well beyond HIV/AIDS:

• We cannot go it alone. Building M&E capacity requires a coordinated approach with other international and national partners and builds on the comparative strengths that each partner brings to the M&E agenda.

• To be sustainable, a long-term commitment to do whatever it takes to support functioning comprehensive M&E systems is necessary. This involves adequate long-term funding and intensive technical support focused on human capacity building and in-country transfer of knowledge and skills.

• To be effective, a focus on sharing lessons learned is essential, not only within countries but also between countries. This requires appropriate knowledge management and regular and transparent communication with national and international partners.

• To sustain enthusiasm in the face of many challenges, we need to not only believe that this can be done but also exert a passion to do it, appropriately guided by a commitment to work collaboratively with and directed by national counterparts.

References

Family Health International. *Behavioral Surveillance Surveys: Guidelines for Repeated Behavioral Surveys in Populations at Risk for HIV.* Arlington, Va.: Family Health International, 2004.

Global Fund to Fight AIDS, Tuberculosis and Malaria. *Annual Report.* Geneva: Global Fund to Fight AIDS, Tuberculosis and Malaria, 2003.

Joint United Nations Programme on HIV/AIDS. *National AIDS Councils: Monitoring and Evaluation Operations Manual.* Geneva: Joint United Nations Programme on HIV/AIDS, 2001.

Joint United Nations Programme on HIV/AIDS. *AIDS Epidemic Update 2003.* Geneva: Joint United Nations Programme on HIV/AIDS, 2003.

MEASURE/ORC Macro. *Guidelines for the Use of HIV Testing in Demographic and Health Surveys.* Washington, D.C.: MEASURE/ORC Macro, 2003.

MEASURE and University of North Carolina. *Strengthening Monitoring and Evaluation of National AIDS Programs in the Context of the Expanded Response.* Chapel Hill: MEASURE, 2002.

National AIDS Commission. *National HIV/AIDS M&E Plan.* Lilongwe, Malawi: National AIDS Commission, 2003.

Office of the U.S. Global HIV/AIDS Coordinator. *The President's Emergency Plan for AIDS Relief: U.S. Five Year Global HIV/AIDS Strategy.* Washington, D.C.: White House, 2003.

World Bank. *Intensifying Action Against HIV/AIDS in Africa: Responding to a Development Crisis.* Washington, D.C.: World Bank, 1999.

World Bank. "Draft Global HIV/AIDS Monitoring and Evaluation Team Strategy Paper [draft]." Washington, D.C.: World Bank, 2003a.

World Bank. *Preparing and Implementing National HIV/AIDS Programs in Africa: The Guidelines and Lessons Learned.* Washington, D.C.: World Bank, 2003b.

World Bank. "Interim Review of the Multi-Country HIV/AIDS Program for Africa: March 2004 [draft]." Washington, D.C.: World Bank, 2004a.

World Bank. "Revised Program Activity Reporting Form [draft]." Washington, D.C.: World Bank, 2004b.

World Bank. "Country Support Team 2004 Progress Report [draft]." Washington, D.C.: World Bank, 2004c.

World Health Organization. *Field Guidelines for HIV Sentinel Surveillance: A Manual for National AIDS Control Programs.* Geneva: World Health Organization, 1999.

DAVID WILSON *is a senior monitoring and evaluation specialist at the World Bank's Global HIV/AIDS Program, Washington, D.C.*

7

In the first three years of Thailand's program, 99 percent of its public hospitals participated in the national monitoring system. Data are used to adjust national or local policies, and practices can be adjusted to improve the program.

Monitoring and Evaluating the National Program to Prevent Mother-to-Child HIV Transmission in Thailand

Siripon Kanshana, Thananda Naiwatanakul,
R. J. Simonds, Pornsinee Amornwichet,
Achara Teeraratkul, Mary Culnane, Nartlada
Chantharojwong, Khanchit Limpakarnjanarat

Thailand has had an epidemic of heterosexually transmitted human immunodeficiency virus (HIV) infection since the mid-1980s that has affected both high-risk populations (such as commercial sex workers) and low-risk populations (such as wives of men who have sex with commercial sex workers). As a result, the prevalence of HIV infection among pregnant women increased from 0 percent in 1990 to about 1.5 percent by 2000 (Kanshana and Simonds, 2002).

Thailand's response to the HIV epidemic has included several successful national HIV-prevention programs. For instance, mandatory screening of all donated blood and eliminating paid blood donors reduced the rate of HIV transmission through blood products to one in eighty thousand transfusions. The national "100 percent condom campaign" that promotes universal use of condoms in commercial sex establishments has substantially increased condom use and decreased HIV and other sexually transmitted infections among young Thai men. Thailand was also the first resource-limited country to implement a national program for preventing mother-to-child transmission (PMTCT) of HIV.

HIV can be transmitted from mothers to their children during pregnancy, at delivery, or through breast-feeding. In Thailand, mother-to-child HIV transmission has already infected thirty thousand children and caused

NEW DIRECTIONS FOR EVALUATION, no. 103, Fall 2004 © Wiley Periodicals, Inc.

seventy-five hundred cases of acquired immunodeficiency syndrome (AIDS) in children. About ten thousand children are born at risk for mother-to-child HIV transmission annually, and without interventions, three thousand children would become infected each year, about one-seventh of all new HIV infections in Thailand (Thai Working Group on HIV/AIDS Projection, 2001).

To address the emerging problem of mother-to-child HIV transmission, the Ministry of Public Health of Thailand in 1993 recommended and began to support routine voluntary HIV testing of women in antenatal care and avoidance of breast-feeding for HIV-infected women (Kanshana and Simonds, 2002). In 1994, a clinical trial in the United States and France demonstrated that a regimen of zidovudine (commonly referred to as *AZT*) given antenatally, intrapartum, and to newborns can reduce the risk of mother-to-child HIV transmission by two-thirds (Connor and others, 1994). Although the use of this regimen was supported for some women in Thailand, it was too complex and expensive to be implemented for all HIV-infected pregnant women.

In 1998, a trial in Bangkok demonstrated that a relatively simple and inexpensive intervention, "short-course" zidovudine, can reduce the risk of mother-infant HIV infection by half among non-breast-feeding HIV-infected women (Shaffer and others, 1999). To gain experience implementing large programs that include short-course zidovudine regimens, pilot programs were supported in two regions of Thailand beginning in 1997–1998 (Thaineua and others, 1998; Kanshana and others, 2000). This was followed by national guidelines in 1999 (Exhibit 7.1) and a national PMTCT program in 2000, the first among resource-limited countries (Kanshana and Simonds, 2002). These guidelines were modified in December 2003 to reflect new research and evaluation findings and new national policy on access to HIV care.

Thailand's Public Health System

Thailand is administratively divided into provinces, districts, and subdistricts; in general, the Ministry of Public Health has a general hospital in each province, a community hospital in each district, and a primary care unit in each subdistrict. In addition, the seventy-six provinces (excluding Bangkok) are grouped into twelve regions, each with at least one regional hospital. Nationwide, there are 25 regional hospitals, 66 general hospitals, 723 community hospitals, and 9,842 primary care units (previously called health centers). All provide antenatal care and are linked by an established network referral system.

Monitoring the National PMTCT Program

To monitor the implementation of its PMTCT program, the Department of Health of the Ministry of Public Health developed a national computerized monitoring system called the Perinatal HIV Implementation Monitoring System (PHIMS) with technical assistance from the U.S. Centers for Disease

Exhibit 7.1. Guidelines for Perinatal HIV Intervention in Thailand (December 1999; modified December 2003)

1. All medical care facilities must have good qualified pre- and post-test counseling for all pregnant women and maintain the blood test results confidentially except for informing the woman and others she gives permission to tell.
2. All pregnant women will be offered voluntary blood testing for HIV antibody using standard methods of the Ministry of Public Health.
3. All HIV-infected pregnant women who decide to continue their pregnancy will be offered zidovudine (AZT) as follows:
   3.1 Start AZT at ~~34~~ 28 weeks' gestation, 300 mg orally every 12 hours.
   3.2 At onset of labor, give nevirapine (NVP) 200 mg and AZT 300 mg orally once and then AZT 300 mg every 3 hours until delivery.
4. For all babies born to HIV-infected mothers, treatment is as follows:
   4.1 When oral fluid can be taken, give single dose of NVP 6 mg (if infant weighs less than 2500 gm, give single dose of NVP 2 mg/kg)
   4.2 Babies born to HIV-infected mothers who got AZT for 4 weeks or more will get AZT syrup 2 mg/kg immediately after birth and continue every 6 hours for 1 week.
   4.3 Babies born to HIV-infected mothers who got AZT for less than 4 weeks will get AZT syrup 2 mg/kg immediately after birth and continue every 6 hours for 6 weeks.
5. All babies born to HIV-infected mothers will get infant formula to substitute for breast-feeding until 12 months of age.
6. All babies born to HIV-infected mothers will get a blood test for HIV antibody at 12 months of age. If the result is positive, the baby will get retested at 18 months of age.
7. ~~Mothers and children who get AZT will get proper medical care and treatment.~~ Mothers and partners will get proper care and will get antiretroviral treatment when clinical definitions are met.
8. Children will get proper care; antiretroviral treatment will be provided for HIV-infected children.

Note: Deletions to the policy in 2003 are indicated by strikethrough, and additions are indicated by underline.

Control and Prevention. PHIMS was designed based on the experience with a monitoring system developed for one of the regional pilot programs, which showed that simple data collection with rapid feedback of program information can help identify and quickly solve problems with program implementation (Kanshana and others, 2000). The original objectives of PHIMS were to monitor the implementation of the national PMTCT program at the hospital level, create a model system for simple and systematic collection and reporting of essential program activities, provide administrative data for resource allocation planning, and provide surveillance data on the prevalence of HIV infection among women in antenatal care.

Data-Collection Instrument. Ministry of Public Health officials at national and local levels, technical consultants, and hospital staff developed a paper-based data collection instrument during a series of meetings (Exhibit 7.2). Because of the large volume of clients in Thailand, it was

Exhibit 7.2. Monthly Report From Mother-to-Child HIV Transmission Prevention Program, Thailand

District: _____   Month of Report: _____

Province: _____   Year of Report: _____

From Antenatal Care (ANC) Clinics

1. Number of women starting ANC   _____ women
   1.1 Number of women who did not have HIV test   _____ women
   1.2 Number of women who had HIV test   _____ women
       1.2.1 Number of women with HIV-positive test   _____ women
       1.2.2 Number of women with HIV-negative test   _____ women

From Delivery Rooms

2. Number of women giving birth   _____ women
   2.1 Number with ANC   _____ women
       2.1.1 Number with positive HIV test   _____ women
             2.1.1.1 Number who took only AZT at least 4 weeks before delivery   _____ women
                     2.1.1.1.1 Number with good compliance   _____ women
                     2.1.1.1.2 Number with fair compliance   _____ women
                     2.1.1.1.3 Number with poor compliance   _____ women
             2.1.1.2 Number who took only AZT less than 4 weeks before delivery   _____ women
             2.1.1.3 Number who took other antiretroviral with AZT   _____ women
             2.1.1.4 Number who took only other antiretroviral, not AZT   _____ women
             2.1.1.5 Number who did not take any antiretrovirals during pregnancy _____ women
       2.1.2 Number with negative HIV test   _____ women
       2.1.3 Number not tested for HIV   _____ women
   2.2 Number without ANC   _____ women
       2.2.1 Number with positive HIV test   _____ women
             2.2.1.1 Number who took only AZT during labor   _____ women
             2.2.1.2 Number who took other antiretrovirals with AZT during labor _____ women
             2.2.1.2 Number who took only other antiretrovirals during labor, not AZT _____ women
             2.2.1.3 Number who did not take antiretrovirals during labor   _____ women
       2.2.2 Number with negative HIV test   _____ women
       2.2.3 Number not tested for HIV   _____ women

3. Number of live births born to women with positive HIV test _____ children
   3.1 Number of children who received only AZT at birth _____ children
       3.1.1 Number of children intending to get AZT for 1 week _____ children
       3.1.2 Number of children intending to get AZT for 6 weeks _____ children
   3.2 Number of children who received other antiretroviral with AZT at birth _____ children
   3.3 Number of children who received only other antiretroviral at birth _____ children
   3.4 Number of children who did not start antiretroviral at birth _____ children
4. Report on formula supply
   4.1 Number of children who received formula before discharge _____ children
   4.2 Amount of formula given to children in 4.1 before discharge _____ . _____ Kg

From Pediatric Clinics
5. Number of children who received formula this month as outpatient _____ children
   5.1 Number of children younger than 1 year who received formula this month _____ children
       5.1.1 Amount of formula used by children in 5.1 _____ . _____ kg
   5.2 Number of children 1–2 years old who received formula this month _____ children
       5.2.1 Amount of formula used by children in 5.2 _____ . _____ kg

feasible to manage only summary information from each hospital each month and not individual patient-level data.

Thus, a data-collection instrument was designed with the following features: summary data that could be derived from log books in each hospital each month; data collected on services provided to women initiating antenatal care, women giving birth, and children born to HIV-infected mothers; a limited number (forty-four) of data elements that would allow monitoring of key program components of HIV testing, provision of antiretroviral medications for preventing mother-to-child HIV transmission (for example, zidovudine), and use of infant formula; and several data items (for example, total number of women tested) that could be calculated and used as internal checks to reduce errors. A two-page report form was printed in Thai on paper that allows two paper copies of different colors to be completed at one time.

Computer System. A computer program was written that includes functions for entry, error checking, compilation, export and import of data, and generation of standard reports. After piloting, the program was compiled onto a compact disk and installed at each provincial health office ($n = 75$), each regional health promotion center ($n = 12$), the AIDS Control Division of the Bangkok Metropolitan Administration, and the Department of Health in Nonthaburi. An operations manual for the computer system was written. A second version of the program was written that allowed for data to be entered at hospitals and imported at provincial health offices.

Data Flow. A system was agreed on for data flow that was implemented in all provinces and Bangkok (Figure 7.1). At the end of each month, each hospital is responsible for completing a monthly report form of data summarized from log books in the antenatal clinic, delivery room, and pediatric clinic, supplemented by data on HIV testing of new antenatal clients at primary care units in the hospital's network. Hospitals can either enter data into this computerized program or send paper reports to provincial health offices for data entry. The provincial health office generates province-level reports and exports provincial data to a file that is sent by electronic mail or diskette to the regional health promotion center. The regional centers import the files from each province, generate region-level user reports, and export their regional data to a file that is sent by e-mail or diskette to the Department of Health. The Department of Health imports the data from each region and generates national-level user reports.

There are nine standard user reports generated at each level of the program: province, region, and national. The standard reports summarize key program indicators by month and relevant geographical area (for example, by hospital for provincial reports) and the number of expected reports that were received.

Training and Supervision. Before implementing the system, a two-day "train the trainers" course was conducted to train responsible staff from each of the twelve regional health promotion centers about how to complete

Figure 7.1. Data Flow for the Perinatal HIV Implementation Monitoring System

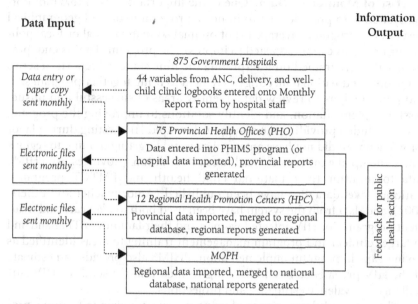

Note: Each region has five to seven provinces. Each province has seven to twenty-two hospitals (one provincial or regional and six to twenty-one community hospitals). ANC, antenatal clinic; MOPH, Ministry of Public Health.

the monthly report forms and use the computer program. Thirty-five people were trained; these regional health promotion center staff then served as regional trainers, consultants in their region, and users of the regional-level program. Each health promotion center then conducted a one- to two-day course for ten to fifteen persons in each province in their region, using a curriculum prepared centrally. The provincial users were taught how to install the program; enter, manage, and export data; and generate the province-level user reports.

Implementation. PHIMS has collected data on services since October 2000. During its first three years (October 2000 to September 2003), 99 percent (866/874) of public hospitals had begun to participate in PHIMS, including hospitals in all seventy-six provinces. Of these hospitals, 647 (74 percent) reported every month and 219 (25 percent) reported some but not all months. Overall, 29,786 (96 percent) of 30,905 expected reports were received during these thirty-six months.

During this period, 1,878,051 (96 percent) of 1,967,250 women who gave birth were tested for HIV, 21,804 (1.2 percent) of women tested were HIV-infected, 16,478 (76 percent) of 21,804 HIV-infected women giving birth received antiretroviral prophylaxis, and 20,105 (94 percent) and

17,838 (83 percent) of the 21,382 children born to HIV-infected women received antiretroviral prophylaxis and infant formula, respectively.

Use of Monitoring Data. One of the important uses of this monitoring system is to provide data to indicate programmatic and geographical areas where program coverage is not optimal so that national or local policies or practices can be adjusted to improve the program. To this end, program staff were trained on interpreting the nine standard reports; a series of regional and national meetings were held to bring together program staff and policymakers to review data, identify areas of successful and unsuccessful implementation, and identify solutions to improving the program. These included providing more support for rapid HIV testing during labor for women who did not have antenatal care and targeting training to regions where the uptake of services was lowest. In addition, provinces use PHIMS data to monitor their maternal child health and PMTCT programs. National-level data also have been published (Amornwichet and others, 2002), and data from the system have been used both to plan care and treatment programs for HIV-infected women and their families in Thailand and to target clinical and program management training to areas identified as having gaps in program implementation. PHIMS also provides an estimate of the HIV prevalence in childbearing women that is useful for HIV surveillance, prevalence estimates, and projections.

This successful experience of using monitoring data to improve programs differs from that of quality improvement methods such as total quality management, which is based on a team-building approach that involves physicians, managers, and staff working together to improve patient care. Implementation of this approach in the United States has had low success rates, in part because it does not allow physicians the autonomy they previously had and threatens established power balances, it has prompted skepticism because of its origins in the private sector, and it has not invested enough time and money in training (Huq and Marin, 2000; Locock, 2003; Trisolini, 2002).

Evaluating the Monitoring System. In 2001, a series of regional meetings of provincial, regional, and national staff were held to evaluate PHIMS; all provinces and regions were represented. Areas of evaluation were functionality of software, barriers to PHIMS implementation, and use of PHIMS data to improve program performance.

About half of hospitals were entering data at the hospital and sending electronic files to the provincial offices. Barriers to hospital data entry identified included frequent change in personnel, high workload and low computer skills of hospital staff, inadequate specifications of hospital computer hardware, frequent use of computers for other functions, computer viruses, and not recognizing the importance of the data for the hospital.

Based on a survey taken during a series of meetings attended by staff from all provinces, fifty-four provinces (72 percent) reported using PHIMS data regularly in presentations to their maternal-child health boards and other venues, and fifty-one (67 percent) reported using PHIMS data to ana-lyze gaps in the PMTCT program. However, sixty-eight provinces (89 per-cent) requested more training in interpreting and using PHIMS data, and seventy (92 percent) expressed the need for guidelines on ongoing moni-toring and supervision for PHIMS. Some provinces reported sending feed-back reports to hospitals; others did not. One region has placed PHIMS data on its regional Web site.

Future Directions for PHIMS. Several new activities are being planned to support and enhance PHIMS:

- Monitoring and supervision guidelines for the national PMTCT program using PHIMS data are being implemented
- Refresher training for PHIMS users, particularly in the aspect of data man-agement, interpretation, and use for improving the PMTCT program, are being implemented
- Software for Web-based entry and reporting is being developed
- Evaluations of data quality and program sustainability are being planned

Evaluating the National Program to Prevent Mother-to-Child HIV Transmission

Because monitoring data are limited in their ability to provide in-depth pro-gram evaluation data, several evaluations of quality, cost, uptake, adherence, and outcomes have been conducted of the PMTCT program in Thailand. In one evaluation of uptake and outcomes, women were interviewed after delivery, and the incidence of infant infections was measured to estimate field effectiveness (Centers for Disease Control and Prevention, 2001). Of the 162 HIV-infected women interviewed, 128 (79 percent) reported hav-ing taken zidovudine. Most women (89 percent) who had taken zidovudine reported not missing any pills. Only 10 women (6 percent) reported having ever breast-fed for a short period. The overall risk for mother-to-child HIV transmission was estimated at 9.6 percent (95 percent confidence interval, 6.4 to 13.5 percent), substantially less than the 25 to 35 percent expected without any interventions.

A tool developed by the Joint United Nations Programme on HIV/AIDS was used to evaluate the quality of counseling and testing in the PMTCT program in two other regions using counseling observation and interviews with women and counselors (Ministry of Public Health of Thailand and World Health Organization, 2000). All sites offered coun-seling before testing, either as a group or individually; all offered individ-ual counseling for women found to be HIV-positive; and most offered counseling and testing during labor and the postnatal periods for women not previously tested. Eighty-two counselors were interviewed in depth about their counseling roles. Most said that they felt comfortable with counseling for PMTCT, but most did not feel valued by their colleagues or supervisors. Only four (5 percent) said they wanted to stop counseling because they found it too stressful.

A cost-effectiveness evaluation of the PMTCT program was done (Teerawattananon and Tangcharoensathien, 2002), which demonstrated that the addition of nevirapine to short-course zidovudine would be expected to be cost beneficial. This regimen has since become national policy.

An evaluation of uptake, adherence, and outcomes was done using postpartum interviews of HIV-infected women giving birth in two large Bangkok hospitals (Chearskul and others, 2002). Of the 448 women who had antenatal care, 350 (78 percent) received zidovudine antepartum; the principal reasons for not receiving zidovudine were lack of information on HIV testing and zidovudine treatment during pregnancy (52 percent) and missed antenatal care appointments (20 percent). One hundred eighteen women (24 percent) did not receive zidovudine during delivery; the principal reasons were precipitous delivery (52 percent) and presenting too late to do a rapid HIV test (37 percent). All 501 infants born to enrolled mothers received zidovudine immediately after birth. The overall mother-to-child transmission rate was 8.6 percent (95 percent confidence interval, 6.2 to 11.6 percent).

Finally, a surveillance system to collect HIV-infection outcomes for children participating in the PMTCT program is currently being piloted in six provinces. This system collects key program information at birth from children born to HIV-infected mothers and then observes children until their HIV-infection diagnosis has been determined at 12 to 18 months of age. The objectives of this pilot system are to determine the rate of mother-to-child HIV transmission on a large population basis, to identify factors associated with continued transmission despite the PMTCT program, to enumerate the number of HIV-infected children for planning purposes, and to evaluate the feasibility of national case reporting of HIV-exposed children for monitoring the effects of the national PMTCT program. The overall mother-to-child transmission rate among 632 children was 6.5 percent (41/632). The rate was 4.6 percent (12/261) among children who had received antiretroviral drugs antenatally, during delivery, and as newborns and 17.6 percent (3/17) among those who had not (Rattanasuporn and others, 2004).

Conclusion

The national program to prevent mother-to-child HIV transmission in Thailand has benefited from a well-utilized national monitoring system that collects information on key program indicators and prepares standard reports that help guide programs at provincial, regional, and national levels. This system not only has helped to track and improve the PMTCT program in Thailand but has been a model for several data systems that are now being implemented in Africa to monitor similar national programs as part of U.S. support through the President's Emergency Plan for AIDS Relief. Similar systems that are simple, user-friendly, and provide useful reports may also be useful for other HIV/AIDS treatment programs.

References

Amornwichet, P., and others. "Preventing Mother-to-Child HIV Transmission: The First Year of Thailand's National Program." *Journal of the American Medical Association,* 2002, *288,* 245–248.

Centers for Disease Control and Prevention. "Evaluation of a Regional Pilot Program to Prevent Mother-Infant HIV Transmission Thailand, 1998–2000." *Morbidity and Mortality Weekly Report,* 2001, *50,* 599–603.

Chearskul, S., and others. "Barriers to Implementing a Short Course Zidovudine Program in Two Bangkok Hospitals, 1999–2001." Barcelona: Fourteenth International Conference on AIDS, July 2002, Abstract WePeB5929.

Connor, E., and others, for the Pediatric AIDS Clinical Trials Group Protocol 076 Study Group. "Reduction of Maternal-Infant Transmission of Human Immunodeficiency Virus Type 1 with Zidovudine Treatment." *New England Journal of Medicine,* 1994, *331*(18), 1173–1180.

Huq, Z., and Marin, T. "Workforce Cultural Factors in TQM/CQI Implementations in Hospitals." *Health Care Management Review,* 2000, *25*(3), 80–93.

Kanshana, S., and others. "Implementing Short-Course Zidovudine to Reduce Mother-Infant HIV Transmission in a Large Regional Pilot Program in Northeastern Thailand." *AIDS,* 2000, *14,* 1617–1623.

Kanshana, S., and Simonds, R. J. "National Program for Preventing Mother-Child HIV Transmission in Thailand: Successful Implementation and Lessons Learned." *AIDS,* 2002, *16,* 953–959.

Locock, L. "Healthcare Redesign: Meaning, Origins and Application." *Quality and Safety in Health Care,* 2003, *12,* 53–57.

Ministry of Public Health of Thailand and World Health Organization. "Evaluation of Voluntary Counselling and Testing in the National Prevention of Mother to Child Transmission Programme in Thailand." 2000. [http://www.unaids.org/publications/documents/health/counselling/JC699-Thai-final-E.doc]. Accessed May 25, 2004.

Rattanasuporn, N., and others. "Result from a Pilot Surveillance System Designed to Determine the Impact of the National Perinatal Prevention Program, Thailand." Bangkok: Fifteenth International Conference on AIDS, July 2004. Abstract ThPeE8058.

Shaffer, N., and others, on behalf of the Bangkok Collaborative Perinatal HIV Transmission Study Group. "Short-Course Zidovudine for Perinatal HIV-1 Transmission in Bangkok, Thailand: A Randomised Controlled Trial." *Lancet,* 1999, *353*(9155), 773–780.

Teerawattananon, Y., and Tangcharoensathien, V. "National Program to Prevent Mother-to-Child HIV Transmission in Thailand: An Analysis of Policy Options." Barcelona: Fourteenth International Conference on AIDS, July 2002. Abstract MoOrF1034.

Thaineua, V., and others. "From Research to Practice: Use of Short Course Zidovudine to Prevent Mother-to-Child HIV Transmission in the Context of Routine Health Care in Northern Thailand." *Southeast Asian Journal of Tropical Medicine and Public Health,* 1998, *29,* 429–442.

Thai Working Group on HIV/AIDS Projection. *Projections for HIV/AIDS in Thailand: 2000–2020.* Nonthaburi, Thailand: Ministry of Public Health, 2001.

Trisolini, M. "Applying Business Management Models in Health Care." *International Journal of Health Planning and Management,* 2002, *17,* 295–314.

SIRIPON KANSHANA is an inspector general and former deputy director of the Department of Health in the Ministry of Public Health in Thailand.

THANANDA NAIWATANAKUL is a senior technical adviser in the Prevention and Care for Families Section at the Thailand MOPH-U.S. CDC Collaboration in Bangkok, Thailand.

R. J. SIMONDS is the chief of the HIV Care and Treatment Branch in the Global AIDS Program of the U.S. Centers for Disease Control and Prevention, Atlanta, Georgia.

PORNSINEE AMORNWICHET is a public health technical officer in the Bureau of Health Promotion of the Ministry of Public Health, Thailand.

ACHARA TEERARATKUL is the chief of the Surveillance and Monitoring and Evaluation Section of the Thailand MOPH-US CDC Collaboration in Bangkok, Thailand.

MARY CULNANE is the chief of the Prevention and Care for Families Section of the Thailand MOPH-U.S. CDC Collaboration in Bangkok, Thailand.

NARTLADA CHANTHAROJWONG is the deputy chief of the Informatics Section of the Thailand MOPH-U.S. CDC Collaboration in Bangkok, Thailand.

KHANCHIT LIMPAKARNJANARAT is the former adjunct director of the HIV/AIDS Collaboration in Bangkok, Thailand.

8

Over 2,500 organizations have been funded to carry out HIV/AIDS interventions in Ghana. A comprehensive and well-coordinated monitoring and evaluation system—one that is simple, strategic, and participatory—is needed to track the national response and its effects.

Planning and Implementing a National Monitoring and Evaluation System in Ghana: A Participatory and Decentralized Approach

Sylvia J. Anie, Emmanuel Tettey Larbi

The current population of Ghana is estimated to be about 20.3 million, with an annual population growth rate of 2.6 percent. The prevalence of human immunodeficiency virus (HIV) infection has remained relatively low and stable, rising from an estimated median of 2.4 percent in 1992 to 3.6 percent in 2003. Substantial variations are found, however, by geographical location, sex, age, and occupation and to a lesser extent by residency (urban versus rural).

The government of Ghana developed, adopted, and is implementing a National HIV/AIDS [Acquired Immunodeficiency Syndrome] Strategic Framework for 2001–2005 (Ghana AIDS Commission, 2000a). This strategic framework recognizes the developmental relevance of the disease and outlines five key domains to prevent and mitigate the socioeconomic effects of HIV/AIDS on individuals, communities, and the nation as a whole. The five key domains are reducing new HIV transmission, providing care and support for people living with or affected by HIV/AIDS, creating an enabling environment, establishing decentralized implementation and institutional arrangements, and conducting research and monitoring and evaluation (M&E).

An Act of Parliament in 2002 established the Ghana AIDS Commission as a supraministerial body under the Office of the President to provide leadership in the coordination of the national response against HIV/AIDS. This position has ensured a high level of political commitment and leadership, which was particularly evident during the design of the national M&E

NEW DIRECTIONS FOR EVALUATION, no. 103, Fall 2004 © Wiley Periodicals, Inc.

framework. As a multisector agency, the Ghana AIDS Commission has the responsibility of advising the government of Ghana in five areas: policy issues relating to HIV/AIDS; formulating strategies, national plans, and guidelines; M&E of the response and its outcomes and effects; advocacy; and mobilizing resources through the active participation of stakeholders. A secretariat serves the Ghana AIDS Commission and implements its decisions and programs. The AIDS commission also established seven technical committees to provide advice on issues such as research, M&E, resource mobilization, legal and ethical matters, prevention and advocacy, project review and appraisal, and care and support including for orphans and vulnerable children.

The multisectoral approach to fighting HIV/AIDS has resulted in an expansion and scaling up of a multiplicity of interventions by civil society and government entities. To date, more than twenty-five hundred organizations have been funded to carry out HIV/AIDS interventions, which has clear implications for M&E (Ghana AIDS Commission, 2000b). Without a comprehensive and well-coordinated M&E system, tracking the national response and its effects is virtually impossible. Such a system should be simple, logical, strategic, and, above all, participatory. In this chapter, we describe the development of a national M&E plan and M&E system for HIV/AIDS in Ghana, based on the National Strategic Framework for HIV/AIDS and the principles of participation and collaboration at community, district, regional, national, and global levels.

Collaborative Process for Developing a National M&E Plan

This section looks at the framework development and capacity assessment for a national M&E plan.

Rationale for a National M&E Plan. M&E is a statutory mandate for the Ghana AIDS Commission. A coherent framework that enables coordination and monitoring of HIV/AIDS activities and their outcomes is essential. A well-designed M&E plan serves four functions. First, it helps to focus the selection of M&E indicators on nationally defined strategic objectives and targets. Second, it guides the systematic collection, processing, and analysis of data at various levels, thus facilitating the coordination role of the Ghana AIDS Commission. Third, it facilitates the standardization of M&E methods and tools across multiple actors at various program levels, ensuring that meaningful comparisons can be made over time. Fourth, it provides the platform for networking partnerships and collaboration among national-level and local-level stakeholders in monitoring and evaluating various components (inputs, activities, outputs, outcomes, and impact) of the national response to HIV/AIDS.

Situational Assessment of M&E Capacity and Systems. To inform the design of an appropriate national M&E plan, a situational appraisal of M&E capabilities, processes, and challenges of stakeholders working in HIV/AIDS was required. Because of the diversity of implementers of HIV/AIDS activities, such as nongovernmental organizations, community-based organizations, faith-based organizations, governmental organizations (ministries, departments, agencies), the private sector, and academic institutions, it was important to ascertain existing M&E systems and skills at each level. The results of this situational analysis, commissioned by the Ghana AIDS Commission in 2002, showed that:

- Partner activities in HIV/AIDS are diverse and numerous, occurring at all levels (that is, community, district, regional, and national).
- M&E capacities and systems are weak in all sectors but particularly in the public sector.
- Fifty-nine percent of implementing organizations do not have an M&E unit, defined as a formalized institutional structure with the sole responsibility of performing M&E. Such an M&E unit would typically consist of M&E experts and data analysis experts.
- Despite not having a formal M&E unit, 65 percent of implementing organizations have a monitoring process in place for tracking their HIV/AIDS activities.
- Most implementing organizations do not have well-defined indicators for HIV/AIDS activities or standardized data-collection instruments. There are generally too many indicators, and they are not harmonized across different organizations.
- Few implementing organizations have baseline data, largely because of the lack of adequate financial resources.
- Different implementing organizations use different indices of program success based on each organization's specific goals.
- Dissemination of M&E information is not carried out on a routine basis.

This study indicated that Ghana would clearly benefit from a comprehensive national M&E plan and framework to ensure the effective coordination and collaboration of the different actors in M&E and to guide the strengthening of their M&E capacity.

Capacity Enhancement for M&E Within the Ghana AIDS Commission. To drive the development process of a national M&E plan while ensuring inclusiveness and multisectoral representation, it was necessary to recruit appropriately trained personnel to the M&E unit within the existing central-level Directorate of Policy Planning, Research, Monitoring, and Evaluation. An M&E specialist and data entry clerks make up the M&E unit. To date, additional expertise in specialist areas such as data analysis and epidemiology has been obtained through outsourcing to contractors, and the capacity of the permanent staff is being enhanced so that eventually they can conduct the necessary M&E activities without extensive external support.

In addition to strengthening the M&E unit, the research, monitoring, and evaluation committee was reorganized and reactivated as a technical committee that would steer the development of the national M&E plan. Careful consideration was given to its membership and to their availability to contribute to the process, balancing skills in M&E with a broad representation of stakeholders. The committee currently comprises representatives from nongovernmental organizations, people living with HIV/AIDS, development partners, ministries (Ministry of Health, Ministry of Food and Agriculture), and academic institutions (University of Ghana, University of Cape Coast). This blend of academia (to ensure a scientific process), development partners (to ensure ownership of the national system and commitment of appropriate financial and technical resources), government agencies (to encourage political ownership), and nongovernmental organizations (to provide lessons learned from existing experiences) formed the bedrock for the success of this committee.

Staff of the Directorate of Policy Planning, Research, Monitoring, and Evaluation and the members of the committee attended several national and international trainings on M&E to strengthen their commitment to M&E and to enable them to share information with counterparts in other countries. During these trainings, the process of developing a national M&E plan was discussed as well as the targets of the United Nations Declaration of Commitment on HIV/AIDS (see Chapter Three, this issue), the Millennium Development Goals (United Nations Development Program, 2004), and the Joint United Nations Programme on HIV/AIDS (UNAIDS) Country Response Information System (see Chapter Six, this issue). The capacity of M&E staff at national, regional, and district levels is continuously being strengthened through their attendance at international and local M&E courses, including trainings organized by the Ghana AIDS Commission. Furthermore, collaboration with development partners and cross-country learning with M&E staff in other countries have encouraged the sharing of knowledge and have further enhanced the capacity of Ghanaian staff.

National M&E Plan. The national M&E plan took six months to develop, which was achieved through a participatory and consultative process (Ghana AIDS Commission, 2003). Agreements were reached regarding appropriate indicators, the type of data sources, and the frequency of data reporting. In addition, participants identified challenges and needs for support. A clear sense of ownership was established through the participatory process and was evident as stakeholders understood the need for their continued involvement over time and offered ongoing logistical, financial, and technical support.

The national M&E plan includes the United Nations Declaration of Commitment indicators as they are relevant to the national epidemic in Ghana, national indicators selected from those recommended by UNAIDS (Joint United Nations Programme on HIV/AIDS, 2000a, 2000b), and country-specific indicators. The selection of the entire set of national indicators was based on the following criteria:

- Relevance to the national HIV/AIDS programs
- Consistency with international standards (the Declaration of Commitment, UNAIDS, the Ghana AIDS Response Fund)
- Sensitivity: ability of the indicator to detect change over time
- Affordability: consideration of data-collection costs
- Usefulness
- Propriety: ethically sound
- Measurability
- Reliability
- Validity

A complete list of national indicators is provided in Table 8.1.

Decentralized Implementation of the National M&E Plan

Over time, Ghana's HIV/AIDS response has begun to focus on decentralization and local community mobilization. Decentralizing the functions of the Ghana AIDS Commission was essential to effectively addressing the complex nature of the determinants of HIV transmission, the geographical variations, and the large number of stakeholders involved in HIV/AIDS activities. In terms of M&E, the benefits of decentralization are that roles and responsibilities can be assigned to different levels, thereby ensuring that the necessary M&E activities are conducted in the most efficient manner. For example, the focus at the national level is on monitoring the overall impact of the various HIV/AIDS programs throughout the country, whereas the regional level takes responsibility for supervising district-led activities. Decentralization requires not only a coherent M&E plan but also the necessary institutional structures to ensure coordination and implementation of M&E activities. Consequently, institutional structures were developed in collaboration with lead agencies, such as the Ministry of Local Government and Rural Development. There are ten regions and 110 districts in Ghana. Each of the ten regions established a regional coordinating council and, within those, ten regional AIDS committees to reflect political mobilization and to provide the necessary administrative and logistical support. The political heads of the regional coordinating councils, the regional ministers, were assigned to be chairpersons of the regional AIDS committees. The core functions of the regional AIDS committees are to monitor the region's local HIV/AIDS activities, establish linkages for cross-regional learning, and integrate best practices in M&E into regional-level policy formulation.

Similarly, district AIDS committees, headed by a district chief executive, were established in each of the 110 districts of the country to coordinate and

Table 8.1. Ghana National Monitoring and Evaluation Indicators

Intervention Areas	Indicators
Prevention of new transmission of HIV	Percentage of adults who are HIV-infected (estimated from data from pregnant women)
	Percentage of pregnant women aged 15 to 24 who are HIV-infected (proxy for HIV incidence)
	Percentage of HIV-infected infants born to HIV-infected mothers
	Percentage of female sex workers who are HIV-infected (estimated from targeted surveillance sites)
Promoting safer sex among the youth and other vulnerable groups	The age at which one-half of young men or young women aged 15 to 24 years have had penetrative sex (median age) of all young people surveyed
	Percentage of women or men aged 15 to 24 who have had sex with more than one partner in the last 12 months
	Percentage of young people aged 15 to 24 reporting the use of condom during sexual intercourse with a nonregular sex partner
	Percentage of young people aged 15 to 24 who both correctly identify ways of preventing the sexual transmission of HIV and reject major conceptions about HIV transmission
	Percentage of respondents who have knowledge of mother-to-child transmission of HIV
	Percentage of schools with teachers trained in life skills-based HIV/AIDS education and who taught it during the last academic year
Prevention and effective management of sexually transmitted infections (STIs)	Percentage of patients with STIs at selected health care facilities who are appropriately diagnosed, treated, and counseled according to national guidelines of all STI patients at those centers
Reduction in blood-borne HIV transmission	Percentage of blood units transfused in the last 12 months that have been adequately screened for HIV according to national or WHO guidelines
Reduction of mother-to-child transmission (MTCT)	Number of centers providing MTCT-prevention services
	Percentage of HIV-infected pregnant women in the last year who are provided with a complete course of antiretroviral therapy to prevent MTCT according to national guidelines
Promoting voluntary counseling and testing (VCT)	Number of centers providing VCT services
	Percentage of people with advanced HIV infection receiving antiretroviral combination therapy
Home-based care for people living with HIV/AIDS	Number of nongovernmental organizations receiving financial assistance from the Ghana AIDS Commission to provide home-based care and support services to people living with HIV/AIDS

Table 8.1. (Continued) Ghana National Monitoring and Evaluation Indicators

Intervention Areas	Indicators
Supportive legal, ethical and policy environment for HIV/AIDS programs	Percentage of women and men aged 15 to 24 who believe that HIV can be transmitted by sharing meals with an infected person
	Percentage of workplaces employing 30 or more people that have HIV/AIDS workplace prevention and care policies and programs
	Percentage of sector ministries with HIV/AIDS work plans and budgets approved and funded by the Ghana AIDS Commission and being implemented
	Number of published reports and HIV/AIDS informational documents distributed to districts
Decentralized implementation and institutional arrangements	Percentage of districts with HIV/AIDS work plans and budgets approved and funded by the Ghana AIDS Commission
	Percentage of all donor funds awarded to community-based organizations in the last 12 months
M&E (monitoring the framework)	Percentage of regions that submit quarterly monitoring reports to the Ghana AIDS Commission
	Number of regional and district focal persons trained in M&E
Research	Number of HIV/AIDS studies endorsed or funded by the Ghana AIDS Commission and disseminated in each of the five intervention areas

WHO: World Health Organization.

monitor district- and community-level HIV/AIDS activities. The district AIDS committees have multisectoral representation and comprise traditional leaders and representatives from faith-based organizations, youth and women's organizations, private organizations, and other organizations operating in the districts.

With such a variety of institutional bodies involved in M&E, the M&E planning process called for an appropriate implementation framework (see Figure 8.1). As illustrated in the figure, the regional AIDS committees and the district AIDS committees provide key functions in M&E to support the Ghana AIDS Commission. A technical team, the District Response Initiative Management Team, operates under the district AIDS committees to provide technical input.

In addition to the formal institutional structures, ten regional and 110 district M&E focal persons were assigned. These are staff of the regional coordinating councils and district committees and represent diverse competencies in planning, monitoring, programming, and budgeting. The roles and responsibilities of the M&E focal persons include the following (Joint United Nations Programme on HIV/AIDS, 2003):

Figure 8.1. National Monitoring and Evaluation Institutional Framework

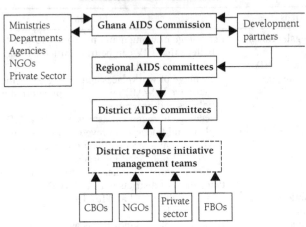

NGOs: nongovernmental organization; CBOs: community-based organizations; FBOs: faith-based organizations.

- Preparing and implementing a regional M&E plan
- Documenting the major activities on HIV/AIDS in the region and preparing quarterly reports for the Ghana AIDS Commission
- Acting as the resource point for information on HIV/AIDS relevant to the region
- Arranging dissemination of information on HIV/AIDS at all levels within the region
- Organizing forums for district M&E focal persons to encourage dissemination of best practices

To encourage their commitment, the M&E focal persons are provided with a monthly allowance. Capacity building and skill development in HIV/AIDS competencies and in M&E are ongoing. In 2003, six training sessions were held for the M&E focal persons, and more trainings are planned for 2004. Ensuring adequate local capacity is imperative if appropriate and competent monitoring of HIV/AIDS activities at the community level is to be achieved.

Work on making the M&E plan operational is continuing, and standardized reporting forms have been developed for four key audiences: ministries, departments, and governmental agencies; nongovernmental organizations; regional coordinating councils and district committees; and private organizations. Reporting procedures are in place at all levels, including for community-based organizations. The institutions referred to in the M&E implementation framework are also those with an interest in the dissemination and use of M&E data. At the national level, there is a large audience for M&E data, including ministries, departments, governmental agencies, private sector groups, trade and labor organizations, professional associations, representative groups of people living with HIV/AIDS, and major nongovernmental organizations. The Ghana AIDS Commission disseminates M&E information widely to ensure that all groups involved in HIV/AIDS activities or with an interest in HIV/AIDS receive relevant information. To facilitate information sharing, the Ghana AIDS Commission has compiled a list of organizations, including contact information and relevant HIV/AIDS intervention areas. At the district level, the primary targets for M&E data dissemination are the district AIDS committees and the district health officers. They receive copies of annual reports and any information from special studies that may be pertinent to their geographical region or their role in the epidemic.

Ongoing Challenges

The decentralization of roles and responsibilities for implementing M&E activities appears to be working, but maintaining the decentralized mechanism is a continuing challenge. Promoting collaboration between the decentralized governmental structures and the national level has been demanding but has been necessary to enhance commitment and ownership. There are still a number of independent vertical reporting systems that do not routinely feed into the district, regional, or national response systems. This is not unexpected because the process of building consensus and trust among partners to share their data takes time and ongoing commitment. The process of consensus building to formalize linkages between the various stakeholders at all levels, therefore, needs to continue to further harmonize reporting systems. In addition, development partners need to be encouraged to feed relevant data into the national M&E system, periodically reporting on the activities they are implementing or funding or both. This is traditionally not a key concern because these agencies are largely interested in M&E for accountability purposes. However, this is now changing with their growing commitment to M&E capacity building in the country. Continued strengthening of M&E capacity is indeed needed, particularly for the M&E focal persons because there is a turnover of trained regional and district M&E focal persons, although attrition is currently not dramatic. The amount of data being received from the regions and districts is substantial and calls into question the capacity of the M&E unit to routinely collate, manage, and analyze the information received. Strengthening of staffing levels or affiliation with external experts will be needed as the national response and its associated M&E system expands.

Conclusion

The Ghana AIDS Commission, all its implementing partners, and the development partners have adopted the national M&E plan as a guideline for M&E at each level. Although challenges continue, Ghana has succeeded in implementing a national M&E system that is sustained by M&E activities at the regional, district, and community levels. Five essential principles have been the basis for this success:

- Dedicated financial resources are available and allocated appropriately for developing M&E units and decentralized structures for M&E.
- The Ghanaian approach has been participatory, with involvement of stakeholders at all levels and consensus building on indicators, key data sources, and reporting procedures.
- Comprehensive planning was done for enhancing existing human resource capacity at all levels, including increasing the understanding of district stakeholders of indicator needs, their use, and their limitations.
- Community, district, regional, national, and global monitoring is linked to a common goal set out in the national M&E plan. This encourages stakeholders to select relevant indicators appropriate to specific needs. Subsets of local indicators are reported to the national level where they are integrated into the national indicator data system.
- Practicality and feasibility are considered, taking into account prevailing challenges and technological drawbacks. The aim has been to develop a simple system with clear lines of responsibility and division of labor.

The current M&E system in Ghana provides a solid basis for further M&E planning and implementation as we learn more about HIV/AIDS; redefine indicators to be more specific, realistic, and measurable; and as we develop new methods for M&E of HIV/AIDS management.

References

Ghana AIDS Commission. *The Ghana National Strategic Framework for HIV/AIDS 2000–2005*. Accra: Ghana AIDS Commission, 2000a.

Ghana AIDS Commission. *A Situational Appraisal of HIV/AIDS Activities in Ghana*. Accra: Ghana AIDS Commission, 2000b.

Ghana AIDS Commission. *A Critical Review and Analysis of Monitoring and Evaluation Systems of Partners Involved in HIV/AIDS Activities in Ghana*. Accra: Ghana AIDS Commission, 2002.

Ghana AIDS Commission. *The National Monitoring and Evaluation Plan for HIV/AIDS in Ghana*. Accra: Ghana AIDS Commission, 2003.

Joint United Nations Programme on HIV/AIDS. National AIDS Councils. *Monitoring and Evaluation Operational Manual*. Geneva: Joint United Nations Programme on HIV/AIDS, 2000a.

Joint United Nations Programme on HIV/AIDS. *National AIDS Programs: A Guide to Monitoring and Evaluation*. Geneva: Joint United Nations Programme on HIV/AIDS, 2000b.

Joint United Nations Programme on HIV/AIDS. *Progress Report on the Global Response to the HIV/AIDS Epidemic, 2003: Follow-Up to the 2001 United Nations General Assembly Special Session on HIV/AIDS*. Geneva: Joint United Nations Programme on HIV/AIDS, 2003.

United Nations Development Program. "The Millennium Development Goals." 2004. [http://www.UNDP.org/mdg]. Accessed June 30, 2004.

SYLVIA J. ANIE is a researcher and director for policy planning, research, monitoring and evaluation at the Ghana AIDS Commission, Ghana.

EMMANUEL TETTEY LARBI is a monitoring and evaluation specialist at the Ghana AIDS Commission, Ghana.

9

Ineffective public health interventions can cost substantial amounts of money that could be directed to more effective programs. The suffering associated with HIV/AIDS necessitates that we proceed with the best possible evidence in hand.

Intervention Research and Program Evaluation: The Need to Move Beyond Monitoring

Greet Peersman, Deborah Rugg

Previous chapters in this issue have mainly focused on issues related to monitoring that allows tracking of program implementation and of trends in the human immunodeficiency virus-acquired immunodeficiency syndrome (HIV/AIDS) epidemic. Although a necessary component of good program management and accountability, monitoring data do not usually provide answers to questions about whether, how, and why a specific program works. More in-depth, systematic inquiry is needed to do this. In this chapter, we focus on the evaluation of HIV-prevention interventions. However, the issues discussed are relevant to other public health interventions and, indeed, the broader field of evaluation. We selected HIV prevention as the area of choice because it is under pressure to prove its effects within a context of competing demands for AIDS treatment that are beginning to scale up around the world. Hence, HIV-prevention evaluation is a pertinent and timely matter.

The advancements in accessibility and efficacy of AIDS treatments must not be allowed to create a false sense of complacency about the continued dangers of HIV infection or to divert attention away from the importance of ongoing prevention efforts (Global HIV Prevention Working Group, 2004). It is not clear whether even the best treatment strategies will be able to contain the virus for an extended period in most HIV-infected individuals or lead to total eradication of the virus. In addition, the general lack of physical, human, and organizational infrastructure in many developing countries slows the implementation of even the relatively simple six-month drug treatment regimens for tuberculosis or the basic immunization of children, let alone the more complex long-term demands of administering complex AIDS drugs (Campbell, 2003). And despite the increased global effort to making AIDS treatment available to those in need, it will take considerable time to reach the estimated 6 million people in need of antiretroviral treatment today (World Health Organization, 2003). Although these biomedical solutions will serve the vital role of alleviating the suffering of many individuals and families in the short term, they will not change the community and social contexts that led to the development of the epidemic in the first place, nor will they strengthen communities in ways that will protect them from future hazards and future epidemics (Campbell, 2003). There is an urgent need for reaffirming our commitment to effective prevention strategies.

Because of the urgency to tackle the HIV/AIDS problem, many prevention programs have rushed to carry out interventions without sufficient grounding in baseline research, models of causality, or lessons learned from small-scale pilot projects. In the haste to mobilize a rapid response, resources for HIV prevention have often been allocated suboptimally, supporting the scaling up of interventions without solid evidence of their effectiveness (Patel, Allen, Keatley, and Jonsson, 2002). This has compromised our ability to control new infections. Around 60 million people have been infected with HIV to date, and about fourteen thousand new infections are occurring daily (Joint United Nations Programme on HIV/AIDS, 2004). Further rises in HIV incidence will be slowed only by massive expansion of prevention efforts. HIV-prevention interventions have maximum potential for impact when they are part of a comprehensive package of interventions and are spearheaded by governments that break the silence around HIV/AIDS and deploy sufficient human and financial resources (Piot, 1999). The effects of these interventions can be enhanced when there are wider public health and development strategies present. Such strategies address the underlying socioeconomic causes that leave people vulnerable to infection and vulnerabilities arising from gender inequalities, the denial of human rights, and discrimination against marginalized groups (Joint United Nations Programme on HIV/AIDS, 2002).

Because the epidemic is constantly shifting, HIV-prevention efforts must continue to be tailored to developments in the epidemic and linked to evaluations that confirm their success or failure (Joint United Nations Programme on HIV/AIDS, 2002). The charge for researchers and program evaluators, then, is to estimate which approaches work best for specific target populations in different epidemiological settings with a given level of inputs in order to allocate resources in a cost-effective manner and for public health practitioners to implement evidence-based interventions (Rehle, Saidel, Mills, and Magnani, 2001).

The body of published literature on interventions in North America and Europe is extensive but is far more sparse for nations in Africa, Asia, and Latin America (Gibney, DiClemente, and Vermund, 1999). Nevertheless, several recent volumes have focused on features of interventions that work or do not work in HIV prevention in developing countries (for example, Cohen and Trussell, 1996; Gibney, DiClemente, and Vermund, 1999; Lamptey and Gayle, 2001; Joint United Nations Programme on HIV/AIDS, 2002; World Bank, 1997). Much less attention has been given to critically analyzing evaluation practices and how they relate to the knowledge base on HIV prevention to date (for example, Gibney, DiClemente, and Vermund, 1999; Oakley, Fullerton, and Holland, 1995; Peersman and Levy, 1998). This chapter fits into the latter category, providing an overview of the current status of intervention research and program evaluations of behavioral HIV interventions, and suggests some pragmatic approaches to improving both evaluation practice and access to evaluation results.

For our purposes, intervention research refers to the implementation of an intervention, often experimental in nature, with the aim of assessing its effects under controlled conditions (that is, an efficacy study). Program evaluation, on the other hand, refers to the assessment of an intervention under real-life conditions (that is, an effectiveness study). We aimed to include both types of studies to obtain a comprehensive overview of evaluation practice to date. We assess the current body of evidence for its credibility and usefulness to making HIV-prevention efforts more effective, guided by the principle of utilization-focused evaluation—evaluation whose purpose is to inform action, enhance decision making, and apply knowledge to solve problems (Patton, 1997).

Finding Outcome Evaluation Studies: Needles in a Haystack

Policymakers, public health practitioners, and researchers need easy access to findings from evaluation reports to guide national policy formulation and strategic program planning, to scale up evidence-based interventions, and to enable the identification of an appropriate research agenda. To obtain a balanced overview of what works and what does not work in HIV prevention, it is essential to locate not only reports that are published in peer-reviewed journals but also those that are part of the "grey" literature. This is important to reduce bias in our judgment of what works because it is well documented that studies reporting on effective interventions are more likely to get published in peer-reviewed journals than those reporting on interventions showing no effect or a harmful effect (Peersman, Oliver, and Oakley, 2001).

In 2002, we conducted an extensive search for evaluation reports published since 1985. We systematically searched three major citation databases (AIDSline, Medline, and PsycLIT), scanned reference lists, contacted relevant researchers and research institutions, and searched Web sites of key HIV/AIDS organizations. Reports were eligible for inclusion if the evaluation focused on assessing the effect of a behavioral HIV prevention on at least one HIV/AIDS outcome (for example, knowledge, attitudes, intentions, behavior, sexually transmitted infections, HIV) *and* the intervention-targeted populations in Africa and Asia. We refer to these studies as outcome evaluations. Behavioral interventions were defined as those aiming to change behavior, either directly or indirectly. These may include individual or group approaches (an individual behavioral component), changing peer or social norms (a social component), administrative or legal changes (a policy component), or structural changes (a structural component, such as changes in health infrastructure or condom provision). Interventions that were biomedical *only* (that is, blood safety interventions, vaccines, prevention of perinatal transmission, microbicides, HIV/AIDS treatment, and sexually transmitted disease treatment) were excluded.

Our search identified more than two thousand citations related to HIV prevention in developing countries, the vast majority describing cross-sectional surveys, case-control studies, cohort studies, discussion papers, reviews, and methods papers. Only 142 citations (7 percent) referred to outcome evaluations of behavioral interventions from Africa and Asia. Locating these outcome evaluations required complex searches, reliable Internet access, access to library services, and a great deal of time. Clearly this is problematic for busy policymakers and public health practitioners, especially in rural areas, who need this information but have limited time to keep up with the literature and often do not have easy access to the Internet or libraries. It is not enough for them to find a few evaluation reports here or there because this may provide a distorted picture of what we know.

One way of ensuring more efficient access to evaluation findings is through support for systematic review efforts such as those the Cochrane Collaboration organizes (http://www.cochrane.co.uk). This is an international, nonprofit, and independent organization dedicated to making up-to-date, accurate information about the effects of health care interventions readily available worldwide. The Cochrane systematic reviews of evaluation research provide an important shortcut to the findings from primary research and assist clinicians, public health practitioners, policymakers, and the general public in making evidence-based decisions. More than twenty reviews on HIV/AIDS prevention, care, and treatment have been disseminated (Institute of Global Health, 2004). The demand for more syntheses is growing as the call for "scientifically based" strategies continues not only in the field of HIV/AIDS but also in other public health and public policy areas. For example, the Campbell Collaboration (http://www.campbellcollaboration.org) was recently established to support systematic reviews that use scientific methods to identify, screen, appraise, and analyze evaluation studies related to education and other social interventions.

Focus of Prevention Outcome Evaluations to Date

To be able to assess what interventions have been evaluated, we developed a systematic coding strategy (Peersman, Flores, and Eke, 2003) to classify the 142 evaluation reports according to key study characteristics: the country

Table 9.1. Characteristics of HIV-Prevention Interventions That Were Evaluated (N = 142)

Characteristic	No. (%)
Nature of intervention	
Individual behavior component	139 (98)
Social component	23 (16)
Policy component	14 (10)
Structural component	12 (8)
Intervention components	
Health education	104 (73)
Health education only	31 (22)
Risk-reduction supplies provision	70 (49)
HIV counseling	41 (29)
Service provision	30 (21)
Skills practicing	23 (16)
Other component(s)	37 (26)
Intervention setting	
Health	36 (25)
Educational	26 (18)
Commercial	19 (13)
Community	17 (12)
HIV/AIDS	14 (10)
Workplace	13 (9)
Outreach	8 (6)
Military	4 (3)
Other setting	33 (23)
Unspecified setting	13 (9)
Intervention provider	
Health care provider	42 (30)
Teacher	15 (11)
Other professional (social worker, lawyer)	44 (31)
Peer	35 (25)
Volunteer	7 (5)
Other provider	37 (26)
Unspecified provider	34 (24)

Note: Columns do not add up to 142 or 100 percent because of multiple categories per study.

where the study was carried out; characteristics of the study population (target, age, sex); the intervention nature (individual behavior, social, policy, structural), intervention components (such as information or skills practicing), intervention site (urban, rural, or transient), intervention setting (for example, community, educational), and the intervention provider (such as health care provider, peer). Table 9.1 summarizes our findings.

Where Have Evaluations Been Conducted, and Who Was Targeted?
Sixty-seven studies (47 percent) were conducted in eighteen different countries in Africa, with Kenya (ten studies), Tanzania (ten), and Zimbabwe (eight) as the top three countries with the highest numbers of evaluation

reports; seventy-five studies (53 percent) were from nine countries in Asia, with Thailand (thirty-six studies), India (fourteen), and the Philippines (four) as the top three. Most of the studies (79 percent) were conducted in urban settings; only 23 percent focused on or included rural settings, and one study focused on a transient setting (a refugee camp). Although the burden of HIV/AIDS in Africa is about tenfold that in Asia and has a much higher level of program activity, this does not seem to be associated with a higher level of evaluation practice (at least not as judged from the number of reports disseminated). In addition, prevention for rural populations, which make up most of the populations in developing countries, and for populations in transient, often high-risk settings seems to be underserved with evaluations. HIV/AIDS has long been viewed as an urban problem, and most attention has been paid to urban areas. However, the number of people living with HIV/AIDS may be greater, in absolute numbers, in rural areas. HIV/AIDS has an additional effect on rural areas because many HIV-positive urban dwellers choose to return to their village of origin when they become ill (Joint United Nations Programme on HIV/AIDS, 2004b). Hence, conducting more evaluations that focus on rural settings is warranted.

Evaluations focused mostly on commercial sex workers (28 percent), clients of HIV testing and counseling services (20 percent), and youth in schools (18 percent). Many fewer studies focused on drug users (8 percent), the military (3 percent), and men who have sex with men (less than 1 percent) as a study population. With a generally high seroprevalence in sex workers around the world, who are at the core of numerous sexual networks, the high focus on evaluation in this group seems appropriate. Female sex workers in developing countries are characteristically poor, have little education, and live in a setting where gender inequality dictates that women have little power within their sexual relationships (Ngugi, Branigan, and Jackson, 1999). Although interventions were mostly focused on individual behavioral components only, an encouraging number of studies with sex workers included social (such as work with brothel owners), structural (such as condom distribution), or policy components (such as 100 percent condom promotion policy in Thailand). Similarly, a focus on youth, who make up almost 50 percent of new cases of infection, is appropriate. However, the argument must be made that youth who are most at risk are not necessarily captured in schools because they drop out of school more often or are less likely to attend in the first place; hence, evaluations with youth also need to address interventions in nonformal settings.

Few studies focused on men who have sex with men, a population highly affected by HIV in Asia (Joint United Nations Programme on HIV/AIDS, 2002), and few studies focused on the military. Because both these groups have been identified as important risk groups (Joint United Nations Programme on HIV/AIDS, 2002), we expected to find more evaluation reports. One explanation is that the development of prevention programs for these population groups has been problematic in many developing countries for reasons of stigma and discrimination (Aggleton, Khan, and Parker, 1999; Haour-Knipe, Leshabari, and Lwihula, 1999). Consequently, the number of intervention research studies is relatively small. Henry (2003) points out that by providing evidence and insight into the problem and its context, evaluation can influence perceptions about social problems, the selection of social policies, and the adaptation of policy implementation. So evaluators should not shy away from conducting evaluations on politically or socially sensitive issues if their work is to contribute to the pursuit of social betterment (Henry, 2000).

What Interventions Were Evaluated? Almost all interventions (98 percent) included an individual behavioral component, but few interventions targeted social, policy, or structural factors that determine the conduciveness of an individual's environment for initiating and maintaining behavioral change. Only 16 percent of interventions included a social component, 10 percent a policy component, and 8 percent a structural component. It has been argued that psychologists, who have dominated the field of HIV prevention, have persistently directed attention toward the individual psychological aspects of sexual behavior and away from the social change that needs to take place to support the likelihood of healthier sexual behaviors (Campbell, 2003; Waldo and Coates, 2000). Social context may play an even bigger role in sexual behavior determination in marginalized communities in less affluent settings than it does for more privileged populations.

Whereas HIV *science* is dominated by behavioral and biomedical research studies informed by narrow psychological theories, the *practice* of HIV prevention has been characterized by a slow but steady shift in the past decade toward more participatory approaches that acknowledge the complex range of determinants of sexual behavior (Campbell, 2003). However, the possibility of learning lessons from such approaches is limited because the move toward more community-oriented interventions has clearly not been matched by evaluation research. For example, a substantial number of interventions (25 percent) used peers to assist with intervention delivery, but only 12 percent of studies focused on the community setting and even less (6 percent) on outreach approaches. In other words, we may possess the most information about the interventions that are least commonly implemented in the context of day-to-day service delivery.

Overall, most interventions took place in formal settings (health care, schools, commercial dwellings, workplace) and used professionals (health professionals, teachers, other professionals such as social workers) to provide the interventions. Because many individuals at highest risk for HIV infection often do not have access to these settings (Joint United Nations Programme on HIV/AIDS, 2002), the lack of studies in informal settings reflects an important gap in our knowledge development.

Interventions typically included health education (73 percent), provision of risk-reduction supplies such as condoms and clean syringes or needles (49 percent), individual or group counseling (29 percent), and provision of services such as treatment of sexually transmitted diseases (21 percent). Almost one in four of the evaluated interventions (22 percent) focused on providing health education *only*, even though it has long been established that knowledge is a necessary but insufficient step for behavioral change (Oakley, Fullerton, and Holland, 1995; Joint United Nations Programme on HIV/AIDS, 2002; World Bank, 1997). On the other hand, the acquisition of relevant risk-reduction skills (such as correct condom use skills, partner negotiation skills) that have been identified as a critical component of effective interventions (Oakley, Fullerton, and Holland, 1995; Joint United Nations Programme on HIV/AIDS, 2002) was rarely addressed. Only 16 percent of interventions included a skills-practicing component. This suggests that new intervention development and associated evaluations may inadequately take into account what we have learned from previous studies. Consequently, time and money have perhaps been wasted on premature evaluations—that is, evaluations of interventions that were insufficiently grounded in behavioral change theory or inadequately developed and hence had little potential to be effective. Evaluations of what can essentially be called "simple" interventions, such as the delivery of health education only, seem insignificant in their contribution to our knowledge base at this stage and should not be prioritized for evaluation or publication.

What Can Be Done? Granted that our search methods, although systematic and extensive, may have missed some relevant studies and that our classification of evaluation reports was necessarily crude, we are confident that we captured a fairly comprehensive view of the intervention research and program evaluation literature. We conclude that many important intervention areas and target populations remain understudied. There are two main reasons: issues of discrimination and marginalization and the fact that evaluation practice lags behind program reality. To tackle these issues, political commitment from the community to the highest political level is required. This makes it possible to bring in all the sectors and players, along with the necessary resources for interventions that address the full need (Piot, 1999). Programs must be guided by a national strategy that is firmly grounded in national realities. Epidemiological surveillance combined with mapping of behavioral risk and socioeconomic vulnerabilities is the best basis for drawing up a national strategy. Subsequently, a countrywide mapping of service availability of what is being done, where, with whom, and with what results is essential to make decisions about expanding program coverage (World Health Organization [http://www.who.org]). The previous chapters in this issue address these important areas of data needs and data collection for monitoring purposes.

A balanced research and evaluation portfolio, then, that addresses relevant national priorities for program implementation and improvement needs to be coordinated by the national AIDS program, rather than by the haphazard interests and capacities of individual researchers and program evaluators. This allows for judiciously using funding for evaluation studies that are relevant to the local context and that address priority needs; identifying who is best placed to design and conduct the evaluation, drawing on local expertise where available; ensuring that resources are commensurate with the evaluation requirements; and requiring a dissemination strategy that is focused on wide and timely dissemination and on the use of the evaluation findings. The last is of particular importance. What is readily available in the public domain tends not to reflect the full extent of evaluations conducted, some of which were never written up or disseminated and some of which were published in local journals or are part of the grey literature that is particularly hard and time-consuming to access. However, what is not available in the public domain cannot contribute to our shared knowledge. The compilation of an inventory of ongoing research and program evaluation, as supported through the Joint United Nations Programme on HIV/AIDS (UNAIDS) Country Response Information System discussed in Chapter Two can facilitate the identification of evaluation needs, the coordination of evaluation studies, and the dissemination and use of research findings.

Barriers to Use of Evaluation Findings

Our analysis indicated that several studies failed to report on key information about the study population and intervention context. For example, the age of the study population was missing in 21 percent of studies, and the sex of the study population was not specified in 6 percent of studies. Twenty-four percent of studies failed to mention the intervention provider; 8 percent did not state whether the study was conducted in an urban, rural, or transient site; and 9 percent did not provide the specific intervention setting (see Table 9.1). Few studies (6 percent) included any indication of costs associated with the implementation of an intervention. The implication of this frequently missing information is that it hinders an assessment of the relevance and applicability of specific study findings to the specific context of those who may be considering replication or scaling up of a specific intervention. Although it is unrealistic to expect that evaluation reports, especially those published in peer-reviewed journals, provide enough detailed information to guide others in the successful replication of an intervention, evaluators must at least be explicit about the study population and the intervention content and delivery. The lack of clear reporting seriously reduces the potential contribution of evaluation research to be used more routinely for improving services. In addition, the fact that virtually none of the studies provided any information related to intervention cost is problematic because cost is an important factor for organizations, especially small community-based organizations, in choosing between alternative effective interventions to support for implementation.

Fortunately, the problem with quality of reporting is something that can be relatively easily resolved. Those writing evaluation reports, as well as peer reviewers and journal editors, can draw on available checklists to ensure that vital information is included in the report, such as "The Consolidated Standards of Reporting Trials (CONSORT)" (Moher, Jones, and Lapage, 2001; Moher, Schulz, and Altman, 2001) and the "Transparent Reporting of Evaluations with Nonrandomized Designs (TREND)" guidelines (Des Jarlais and others, 2004). In addition, Grob (2003) identified inherent qualities of a good evaluation report that increases the potential for decision makers to use the evaluation findings. A useful report provides contextual information that allows the readers to put things in perspective; it presents persuasive evidence that is both strong and relevant, and therefore the findings are compelling; and it includes recommendations geared for impact—things that program managers and policymakers can actually do, can afford to do, and that, if done, will achieve results (Grob, 2003).

What Is the State of the Science in Evaluation Practice?

In addition to categorizing the evaluation reports by intervention and study population characteristics, as discussed above, details of the study design and execution were noted: the number of intervention groups involved in the study, sample size, attrition rates and reporting of characteristics of dropouts, types of outcomes measured and time interval for measurements, and inclusion of process measures. Studies were also assessed for the presence or absence of four methodological quality criteria: baseline equivalence between the intervention and comparison-control groups, reporting of baseline outcome measures, reporting of postintervention outcome measures, and reporting on all outcomes that the intervention targeted to change. First of all, our focus on multiple group designs is grounded in the well-established fact that estimates of effectiveness are considerably higher in outcome evaluations that lack a control or comparison group than in well-designed experimental and quasi-experimental studies (Oakley, 2001). Second, it is important to establish that people who make up the control or comparison group have similar characteristics to those in the intervention group. If they do not, then any differences between them following the intervention may be due to preexisting inequalities, leading to erroneous conclusions about the effectiveness of the intervention. Third, reporting both baseline and follow-up outcome measures is essential to obtain a clear understanding of the magnitude of the intervention effects. And, last but not least, insisting on reporting of all outcomes targeted for change by the intervention is important in fully understanding the worth of an intervention. Often, interventions are designed with the aim to change knowledge, attitudes, intentions, and behavior, but evaluation reports frequently fail to report on the full range of outcome measures, guided by the desire to report

Figure 9.1. Outcomes Measured in Evaluations of HIV-Prevention Interventions (N = 142)

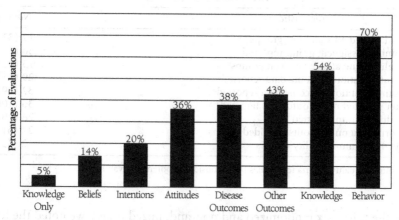

on positive rather than negative or no effects (adding to the publication bias discussed above). Studies meeting all four quality criteria were deemed to have adequate methodological rigor for the evaluation findings to be considered potentially valid. (Other issues related to execution, data analysis, and interpretation would then need to be taken into account, but these are outside the scope of this article.) The implication for studies not exhibiting these criteria is that the effect of the intervention tested is unknown at this stage and would need to be subjected to additional evaluation if addressing a pertinent program need. The approach used in these methodological reviews follows the model for reviewing the effectiveness of health care interventions established within the Cochrane Collaboration and the work of other reviewers in the health education and social welfare fields (Peersman, Oakley, and Oliver, 1999). Admittedly, these are stringent review criteria for which the Cochrane method is known. Because methodological reviews of HIV-prevention interventions have been lacking, we thought it was important to at least use the well-established Cochrane approach to reviewing the existing literature because so much is at stake. Our findings are summarized in Figure 9.1 and Table 9.2.

The vast majority of studies (75 percent) used a one-group design (lacking a control or comparison group) but typically included both preintervention and postintervention outcome assessments. Multiple group designs (referred to as trials) used random allocation to groups (randomized trials) in 8 percent and a nonrandom method in 17 percent of studies. Most studies assessed a range of outcomes, including behavioral measures (70 percent) and disease outcomes (38 percent) (see Figure 9.1).

Looking in more detail at the methodological quality of the evaluations employing a multiple group design (that is, these issues were assessed only

**Table 9.2. Characteristics of Trials of HIV Prevention
Interventions (n = 36)**

Characteristic	No. (%)
Randomized allocation to groups	12 (33)
Numbers assigned; group reported	36 (100)
Baseline equivalence between groups[a]	15 (42)
Preintervention outcome data reported[a]	29 (81)
Postintervention outcome data reported[a]	32 (89)
Data reported on all outcomes targeted[a]	36 (100)
Attrition/group reported	28 (78)
Information on dropouts provided	22 (61)
Met 4 minimum quality criteria[a]	12 (33)

[a]Minimum quality criteria for studies to be considered potentially valid.

for the thirty-six randomized and nonrandomized trials), we noted the following: more than 75 percent (twenty-seven) of all trials reported essential information related to sample size, attrition rates, preintervention and postintervention outcome data, and data on all targeted outcomes. However, information on those who dropped out of the study and therefore were unavailable for follow-up measurement was less commonly reported (61 percent, or twenty-two). In addition, only a third of all trials (thirteen) met *all* four quality criteria, with the implication that the conclusions about effectiveness presented by the authors cannot be treated as valid. Despite these methodological challenges, the authors of eighteen trials (50 percent) concluded that the intervention resulted in positive changes in the outcomes targeted, the authors of twelve trials (33% percent indicated a mixed effect (positive effect for some outcomes only), and the authors of six trials (17 percent) stated that the intervention was ineffective.

On the upside, it is encouraging to see that fairly large sample sizes were used in trials, ranging from 84 to 5,657 individuals, with more than half of the trials (58 percent, or twenty-one) including more than 500 individuals in the study; and individuals were observed for relatively long periods, ranging from immediately after completion of the intervention to three years after intervention, with sixteen trials (44 percent) including at least a six-month follow-up assessment and twelve trials (33 percent) one year or more.

Probably of greatest concern is the paucity of methodologically sound evaluations. The vast majority of studies (91 percent, or thirty-three) were considered to provide inconclusive evidence due to a number of reasons: lack of inclusion of a control or comparison group (75 percent [twenty-seven]); significant differences between groups at baseline in terms of outcome measures targeted (including some of the randomized trials) (58 percent [four]); and failure to report preintervention, or postintervention, or both, outcome measures (19 percent [seven] and 11 percent [one], respectively). With these limitations, the findings from such evaluations should be seen as suggestive, or at best plausible, but certainly not proved.

Although it may appear that we are preoccupied with small methodological issues that the field of evaluation has addressed literally for decades, these do have policy implications. Public health interventions can, indeed, do harm as well as good, and even when they have no effect could cost substantial amounts of money that could be directed to more effective interventions. The huge opportunity cost (money could be better spent elsewhere) and the suffering associated with HIV/AIDS necessitates the need for effective HIV prevention, and we must proceed with the best possible evidence in hand. These are all good reasons why well-designed outcome evaluations have a place in HIV prevention. Over the years, several researchers have argued the urgent need for a commitment to funding the careful design and evaluation of HIV-prevention interventions (for example, Bollinger, Cooper-Arnold, and Stover, 2004; Coyle, Boruch, and Turner, 1991; Oakley, Fullerton, and Holland, 1995; Peersman and Levy, 1998). Although high-quality evaluation research is often costly, uncertainty about program effectiveness is even more costly, as Coyle, Boruch, and Turner in 1991 (p. vii) pointed out: "The price of ignorance will be measured both in dollars spent on ineffective programs and in deaths and disease that might have been prevented."

On the one hand, program evaluation as a field has viewed responsiveness to a particular stakeholder or stakeholders as an important attribute to increase use of evaluation findings, sometimes at the cost of technical quality (Patton, 1997). On the other hand, scientists have argued that if evaluation findings are dismissed because of technical flaws or mired down by squabbles over their accuracy, it is unlikely that they will be influential in terms of their contribution to the social good (Henry, 2003). Indeed, Ginsburg and Rhett (2003) defined a useful evaluation as one that adds to the body of timely, relevant evidence to increase the likelihood that policy decisions improve program performance. They refer to recent U.S. federal legislation creating the Institute for Education Sciences and requiring evaluation designs that allow for the strongest possible causal inferences, including randomized, controlled trials. Surely, the standards should not be different for public health interventions in developing countries. However, we need to look at what rigor criteria are to be adhered to for testing interventions within research conditions versus applied programmatic settings. (In our analysis, we applied the same criteria to both.) Bryce and others (2004) argue that few public health programs are implemented in ways that can support evaluations that are either entirely "efficacy" or entirely "effectiveness" and that this dimension of evaluation should be considered as a continuum. The criteria for rigor may therefore be not so much related to the setting but rather to the level of uncertainty about the intervention and the importance of its potential application.

The need for rigorous outcome evaluation does not, of course, mean that other types of research and evaluation are not relevant or, indeed, essential for answering critical questions (Oakley, 2001; Victora, Habicht, and Bryce, 2004). For starters, there is a need for better integration of process and outcome evaluation. Only about a third of studies (32 percent) included process measures (such as measures related to the quality of intervention materials and intervention implementation, and client satisfaction with provided services). Yet, as thirty years of evaluation literature affirms, examining outcomes without assessing whether the intervention was implemented as planned could also lead to erroneous conclusions regarding the effect of the intervention (Rehle, Saidel, Mills, and Magnani, 2001).

In addition, complementary methods for conducting evaluation and for analyzing evaluation findings need to be further explored and more systematically developed (Bryce and others, 2004; Victora, Habicht, and Bryce, 2004). Ginsburg and Rhett (2003) suggest several approaches in addition to rigorous evaluations to build a better body of evidence to strengthen evaluation use. First is the potential for performing rigorous syntheses of relevant research and evaluations that can support program improvement by cumulating bodies of evidence across many small, rigorous studies focused on a particular intervention approach. There are several examples where systematic reviews have been successfully used, and several efforts to undertake such reviews are already underway (the Cochrane and Campbell collaborations mentioned earlier). Second, we can develop scientifically sound, large-scale databases that are particularly suited to address important descriptive, rather than causal, programmatic questions. These databases should contain intervention and service descriptions and key outcome variables from cross-sectional or longitudinal samples in large-scale surveys. A third additional method is conducting well-designed case studies to gather in-depth information that is not possible to collect through broad surveys. A case-study method can be used to help identify problems with program implementation, suggest ways for designing effective practices, and help refine research questions and tools (Ginsburg and Rhett, 2003).

Another approach that is often mentioned but that remains ill defined is triangulation. There are basically two kinds: checking out the consistency of findings generated by different data-collection methods, and checking out the consistency of different data sources within the same method. The aim of triangulation is verification from different angles, but when triangulation is applied in practice, we often find that data from different sources or collected using different methods may conflict (Oakley, 2000). The basic premise of triangulation is a good one because our data sources need to be inclusive and our evaluation methods need to be varied, both contributing to a more comprehensive picture of "reality." But we need to find better ways to plan intentionally for comprehensiveness, and we need to understand when it is vital. We also need to develop explicit and well-rationed approaches for analyzing and interpreting (triangulating) the results obtained. An important example of a comprehensive yet strategic evaluation is provided by Bryce and others (2004) in the multicountry evaluation of an integrated program for improving child health and development. The methodological insights gained by this study can contribute to the development and refinement of methods for conducting large-scale evaluations of public health interventions in general and HIV/AIDS interventions in specific.

Conclusion

To increase access to the evaluation literature and to improve the quality and breadth of evaluation research and program evaluation, program managers, evaluator-researchers, evaluation funders, and journal editors need to undertake a concerted effort.

Program Managers

- Plan for evaluation up front and not as an afterthought, which would reduce the risk of unanticipated, but often preventable, problems

Evaluator-Researchers

- Work within the priorities set by local governments and communities
- Allow adequate time for intervention development before undertaking evaluation and to evaluate implementation processes as well as intervention effects
- Be knowledgeable about how best to draw on existing data sources and the use of a combination of qualitative and quantitative methods to provide a richer interpretation of the lessons learned from HIV-prevention efforts
- Explicitly document all methods and findings and take responsibility for wide dissemination of the evaluation report in a timely manner

Funders

- Provide guidance on evaluation methods that match evaluation questions
- Apply selection procedures that favor studies that fill important knowledge gaps
- Provide adequate resources to support full implementation of sound evaluations and facilitate dissemination

Journal Editors

- Apply standardized and stringent peer-review procedures that assess both the adequacy of reporting and the methodological limitations of the evaluation study so that those studies that make a substantial contribution to our knowledge base receive priority for publication

Analyses like the ones presented in this chapter are sometimes greeted with "this is known, what's new?" We do, indeed, hope that we are preaching to the converted. Evaluators around the world are moving good evaluation practice forward, but our analysis is a reminder that we have not yet arrived. We should be ever-vigilant and open to new ideas and alternative ways of doing things. Applying a range of methods in a well-reasoned manner to priority issues, informed by what we know from previous evaluations, will help us contribute critical knowledge to improving the effectiveness of the fight against HIV/AIDS.

References

Aggleton, P., Khan, S., and Parker, R. "Interventions for Men Who Have Sex with Men." In L. Gibney, R. DiClemente, and S. Vermund (eds.), *Preventing HIV in Developing Countries: Biomedical and Behavioral Approaches.* New York: Kluwer/Plenum, 1999.

Bollinger, L., Cooper-Arnold, K., and Stover, J. "Where Are the Gaps? The Effects of HIV-Prevention Interventions on Behavioral Change." *Studies in Family Planning,* 2004, *35,* 27–38.

Bryce, J., and others. "The Multi-Country Evaluation of the Integrated Management of Childhood Illness Strategy: Lessons Learned for the Evaluation of Public Health Interventions." *American Journal of Public Health,* 2004, *94*(3), 406–415.

Campbell, C. *"Letting Them Die": Why HIV/AIDS Prevention Programs Fail.* Bloomington: Indiana University Press, 2003.

Cohen, B., and Trussell, J. (eds.). *Preventing and Mitigating AIDS in Sub-Saharan Africa: Research and Data Priorities for the Social and Behavioral Sciences.* Washington, D.C.: National Academy Press, 1996.

Coyle, S., Boruch, R., and Turner, C. (eds.). *Evaluating AIDS Prevention Programs.* (Exp. ed.) Washington, D.C.: National Academy Press, 1991.

Des Jarlais, D., Lyles, C., Crepaz, N., and the TREND Group. "Improving the Reporting Quality of Nonrandomized Evaluations of Behavioral and Public Health Interventions: The TREND Statement." *American Journal of Public Health,* 2004, *94*(3), 361–366.

Gibney, L., DiClemente, R., and Vermund, S. (eds.). *Preventing HIV in Developing Countries: Biomedical and Behavioral Approaches.* New York: Kluwer/Plenum, 1999.

Ginsburg, A., and Rhett, N. "Building a Better Body of Evidence: New Opportunities to Strengthen Evaluation Utilization." *American Journal of Evaluation,* 2003, *24*(4), 489–498.

Global HIV Prevention Working Group. "HIV Prevention in the Era of Expanded Treatment Access." 2004. [http://www.gatesfoundation.org]. Accessed June 30, 2004.

Grob, G. "A Truly Useful Bat Is One Found in the Hands of a Slugger." *American Journal of Evaluation,* 2003, *24*(4), 499–505.

Haour-Knipe, M., Leshabari, M., and Lwihula, G. "Interventions for Workers Away From Their Families." In L. Gibney, R. DiClemente, and S. Vermund (eds.), *Preventing HIV in Developing Countries: Biomedical and Behavioral Approaches.* New York: Kluwer/Plenum, 1999.

Henry, G. "Why Not Use?" In V. Caracelli and H. Preskill (eds.), *The Expanding Scope of Evaluation Use.* New Directions for Evaluation, no. 88. San Francisco: Jossey-Bass, 2000.

Henry, G. "Influential Evaluations." *American Journal of Evaluation,* 2003, *24*(4), 515–524.

Institute of Global Health. "Cochrane Review Group on HIV infection and AIDS." 2004. [http://www.igh.ucsf.edu/program_activities/cochrane_collaborative_review.html]. Accessed June 30, 2004.

Joint United Nations Programme for HIV/AIDS. *Report on the Global HIV/AIDS Epidemic.* Geneva: Joint United Nations Programme for HIV/AIDS, 2002.

Joint United Nations Programme for HIV/AIDS (UNAIDS). "About 14,000 New HIV Infections a Day in 2003." 2004a. [http://www.UNAIDS.org/Bangkok2004/report_pdf.html.] Accessed June 30, 2004.

Joint United Nations Programme for HIV/AIDS (UNAIDS). "Rural HIV/AIDS: Fact Sheet." 2004b. [http://www.UNAIDS.org]. Accessed June 30, 2004.

Lamptey, P., and Gayle, H. (eds.). *HIV/AIDS Prevention and Care in Resource-Constrained Settings: A Handbook for the Design and Management of Programs.* Arlington, Va.: Family Health International, 2001.

Moher, D., Jones, A., and Lapage, L. "Use of the CONSORT Statement and Quality of Reports of Randomized Trials: A Comparative Before-and-After Evaluation." *Journal of the American Medical Association,* 2001, *285,* 1992–1995.

Moher, D., Schulz, K., and Altman, D. "The CONSORT Statement: Revised Recommendations for Improving the Quality of Reports of Parallel-Group Randomized Trials." *Lancet,* 2001, *357,* 1191–1194.

Ngugi, E., Branigan, E., and Jackson, D. "Interventions for Commercial Sex Workers and Their Clients." In L. Gibney, R. DiClemente, and S. Vermund (eds.), *Preventing HIV in Developing Countries: Biomedical and Behavioral Approaches.* New York: Kluwer/Plenum, 1999.

Oakley, A. *Experiments in Knowing: Gender and Method in Social Sciences.* Cambridge, U.K.: Polity Press, 2000.

Oakley, A. "Evaluating Health Promotion: Methodological Diversity." In S. Oliver and G. Peersman (eds.), *Using Research for Effective Health Promotion.* Bristol, Pa.: Open University Press, 2001.

Oakley, A., Fullerton, D., and Holland, J. "Behavioral Interventions for HIV/AIDS Prevention." *AIDS,* 1995, *9,* 479–486.

Oakley, A., and Oliver, S. "Looking to the Future: Policies and Opportunities for Better Health." In S. Oliver and G. Peersman (eds.), *Using Research for Effective Health Promotion.* Bristol, Pa.: Open University Press, 2001, pp. 183–184.

Patel, M., Allen, K., Keatley, R., and Jonsson, U. "Introduction." *Evaluation and Program Planning,* 2002, *25,* 317–327.

Patton, M. Q. *Utilization-Focused Evaluation.* (3rd ed.) Thousand Oaks, Calif.: Sage, 1997.

Peersman, G., Flores, S., and Eke, A. *Systematic Review on Interventions for Preventing HIV-Infection in Developing Countries: Coding Rules for Bibliographic Register.* Atlanta: Monitoring and Evaluation Team, Global AIDS Program, Centers for Disease Control and Prevention, 2003.

Peersman, G., and Levy, J. "Focus and Effectiveness of HIV-Prevention Efforts for Young People." *AIDS,* 1998, *12*(suppl. A), S191–S196.

Peersman, G., Oakley, A., and Oliver, S. "Evidence-Based Health Promotion? Some Methodological Challenges." *International Journal of Health Promotion and Education,* 1999, *37,* 59–64.

Peersman, G., Oliver, S., and Oakley, A. "Systematic Reviews of Effectiveness." In S. Oliver and G. Peersman (eds.), *Using Research for Effective Health Promotion.* Bristol, Pa.: Open University Press, 2001.

Piot, P. "Foreword." In L. Gibney, R. DiClemente, and S. Vermund (eds.), *Preventing HIV in Developing Countries: Biomedical and Behavioral Approaches.* New York: Kluwer/Plenum, 1999.

Piscine, E., and others. "Back to Basics in HIV Prevention: Focus on Exposure." *British Medical Journal,* 2003, *326,* 1384–1387.

Rehle, T., Saidel, T., Mills, S., and Magnani, R. "Conceptual Approach and Framework for Monitoring and Evaluation." In T. Rehle, T. Saidel, S. Mills, and R. Magnani (eds.), *Evaluating Programs for HIV/AIDS Prevention and Care in Developing Countries: A Handbook for Program Managers and Decision Makers.* Arlington, Va.: Family Health International, 2001.

Victora, C., Habit, J., and Bryce, J. "Evidence-Based Public Health: Moving Beyond Randomized Trials." *American Journal of Public Health,* 2004, *94*(3), 400–405.

Waldo, C., and Coates, T. "Multiple Levels of Analysis and Intervention in HIV Prevention Science: Examples and Directions for New Research." *AIDS,* 2000, *14*(suppl. 2), S18–S26.

World Bank. *Confronting AIDS: Public Priorities in a Global Epidemic*. New York: Oxford University Press, 1997.

World Health Organization. *Treating 3 Million by 2005: Making It Happen. The WHO Strategy*. Geneva: World Health Organization, 2003.

GREET PEERSMAN *is the technical deputy director of the Monitoring and Evaluation Team for the Global AIDS Program at the U.S. Centers for Disease Control and Prevention, Atlanta, Georgia.*

DEBORAH RUGG *is the associate director of the Monitoring and Evaluation Team for the Global AIDS Program at the U.S. Centers for Disease Control and Prevention, Atlanta, Georgia.*

10

National monitoring and evaluation systems are failing to gather basic information. Too many data are being collected for various donors for their exclusive accountability purposes.

Global Standards for Monitoring and Evaluating National AIDS Programs: Challenges, Concerns, and Needs of Developing Countries

Nicolas Meda

Today more than 40 million people live with human immunodeficiency virus-acquired immunodeficiency syndrome (HIV/AIDS) worldwide, and nearly 80 percent of them live in developing countries. Each day, the twelve thousand new HIV infections occurring in the developing world relentlessly weigh down the already-heavy burden it endures in this pandemic. Containing the spread of HIV is one of the greatest challenges developing countries will face during this millennium.

In addition to conflicts, population displacements, labor migration, decaying national health systems, unsafe sex, and poverty, De Lay and Manda (Chapter One) suggest several other factors that could explain the disastrous situation of the HIV/AIDS epidemic in developing countries. One of them is the denial of the epidemic's magnitude by many national governments anxious to develop their tourist industries. Another factor is the difficulty many countries face in building an appropriate national response within the context of social, cultural, religious, and political values fueling the stigmatization and discrimination of people living with HIV/AIDS. A third factor is the lack of political will and the insufficient resources that have not made it possible to match the global response with the magnitude of the epidemic. Finally, as Peersman and Rugg point out (Chapter Nine), in places where people have acted, many of the scarce resources were wasted on the implementation of inappropriate programs of unknown effectiveness.

NEW DIRECTIONS FOR EVALUATION, no. 103, Fall 2004 © Wiley Periodicals, Inc.

Nowadays many suggest that the world is at an unprecedented turning point in the fight against HIV/AIDS. We have more resources; more robust interventions in HIV/AIDS prevention, treatment, and care; and more experience and "know how." Governments in almost all developing countries now have multisector national AIDS control programs and are implementing strategies that key international policymakers recommend.

There has been a consensus for a long time that it is absolutely unethical to implement interventions of unknown efficacy or cost-effectiveness (Lin and Gibson, 2003). Thus, it is the role of intervention research to contribute to generating robust evidence on HIV/AIDS programs (Habicht, Victora, and Vaughan, 1999). Monitoring and evaluation (M&E), as posed by Øvretveit (2002), then plays a role during the implementation of an efficacious program. M&E examines whether the program is implemented as planned and according to the quality standards agreed upon, whether it applies knowledge to solve problems, and whether it makes the necessary programmatic changes. M&E measures program success, ensures accountability, and directs resources to achieve maximum public health effects.

Because of the involvement of many donors, agencies, institutions, and organizations at the country level, it is difficult to attribute any success or failure to a specific HIV/AIDS program. Instead, it is our common responsibility to achieve collective effectiveness in controlling the HIV/AIDS epidemic within the multisector national HIV/AIDS program. To do that, the United Nations General Assembly Special Session Declaration of Commitment on HIV/AIDS has put pressure on countries to accelerate program implementation, scale up interventions, and report on achievements against predefined targets (see Chapter Three).

Chapter Two on global advances in M&E reminds us of the progress made in M&E over the years, from the era of AIDS reporting with the Bangui definition in 1985, to HIV sentinel surveillance conducted since 1987, the first priority prevention indicators defined in 1994, and the move toward implementation of second-generation surveillance since 1998. In 2000, an international partnership permitted us to develop what we can call the global standards in M&E of national AIDS programs (Joint United Nations Programme on HIV/AIDS, 2000), now complemented with additions focused on specific program areas (see Chapter Five).

Many countries have used these toolkits to develop and implement their national M&E plan. Thailand offers an example of a functioning M&E system for the national program for preventing mother-to-child transmission of HIV (see Chapter Seven). A national monitoring system with limited data elements, coupled with ongoing technical and financial support, was successfully implemented and has proved useful for improving the program in Thailand. However, from the process in Ghana, we have learned that often there are too many persistent independent vertical reporting systems that do not feed into district, regional, and national responses (see Chapter Eight). The same is true in many other countries, where the Global Fund to Fight

AIDS, Tuberculosis and Malaria and the World Bank Multi-Country AIDS Program (see Chapter Six), the World Health Organization/Italian AIDS Initiative, the Centers for Disease Control and Prevention's Global AIDS Program, and others all have their own M&E plan at the country level.

We are now moving toward the development of a global organizing framework, harmonized indicators, a coordinated approach to capacity building, and the implementation of a unified national M&E system that takes into account local experience and global expertise (see Chapter Two). Partnerships, communication, knowledge sharing, coordination, and collaboration are key values and successful mechanisms to achieve our goals in M&E. The U.S. Agency for International Development and the Centers for Disease Control and Prevention are piloting these mechanisms in their target countries in the developing world (see Chapter Four).

However, the reality from the field is not so optimistic. National M&E systems are not gathering even the most basic information to improve the day-to-day implementation of HIV/AIDS programs. At the country level, too many different data need to be collected for various donors for their exclusive accountability purposes. As a participant of one UNAIDS workshop devoted to M&E capacity strengthening in developing countries noted, "An epidemic of indicators has spread, and most international agencies and donors are now infected." As a result, data are not necessarily being used for policy and program improvement (see Chapter Three). In Ghana, the lack of M&E capacity at the National AIDS Council Secretariat and the difficulty of involving and adequately using relevant national experts from other institutions remain a big challenge (see Chapter Eight). As a matter of fact, this situation is common in the majority of developing countries.

The challenges for M&E in the field are twofold: there is a multiplicity of players for M&E capacity strengthening, and a sustainable plan to develop autonomous human resource capacities at the country level is lacking. It is difficult to count on workshops only to develop a national capacity for M&E. In addition to various models of training, the use of best practices in management, enhanced working environments, logistics support, staff motivation, and control for accountability must also be integrated parts of capacity strengthening for M&E in developing countries. In this context, the "three ones" principle, introduced by UNAIDS (see Chapter Two), offers a glimmer of hope for developing countries to capitalize on all the resources and expertise of the various stakeholders and in-country players to feed their national AIDS program M&E systems and, if possible, only one national M&E system per country.

References

Habicht, J., Victora, C., and Vaughan, J. "Evaluation Designs for Adequacy, Plausibility and Probability of Public Health Program Performance and Impact." *International Journal of Epidemiology*, 1999, *28*, 10–18.

Joint United Nations Programme on HIV/AIDS. *National AIDS Programs: A Guide to Monitoring and Evaluation.* Geneva: Joint United Nations Programme on HIV/AIDS, 2000.

Lin, V., and Gibson, B. *Evidence-Based Health Policy: Problems and Possibilities.* New York: Oxford University Press, 2003.

Øvretveit, J. *Action Evaluation of Health Programs and Changes: A Handbook for a User-Focused Approach.* Oxon, U.K.: Radcliffe Medical Press, 2002.

NICOLAS MEDA *is a Medical epidemiologist and senior researcher at the Centre MURAZ/Ministry of Health, Burkina Faso.*

11

The challenges ahead are at least as daunting as those already overcome: demonstrating that monitoring and evaluating findings can make a difference in the lives of people.

A Microcosm of the Global Challenges Facing the Field: Commentary on HIV/AIDS Monitoring and Evaluation

Michael Quinn Patton

Stake (2004), in a provocative and insightful article, asks "How Far Dare an Evaluator Go Toward Saving the World?" He identifies six advocacies common in evaluation studies. I want to use his framework to position this review and commentary. (The direct quotations in the six items are from Stake, 2004, p. 104.)

1. *We often care about the thing being evaluated.* Stake was one of the first evaluation theorists to clearly articulate that we do not have to pretend neutrality about the problems programs are attacking to do fair, balanced, and neutral evaluations of those programs. Who wants an uncaring evaluator who professes neutrality about homelessness, hunger, child abuse, or community violence?

I care about human immunodeficiency virus-acquired immunodeficiency syndrome (HIV/AIDS). My younger brother died of AIDS early in the epidemic. My entire family has been involved actively in AIDS Walks and other activities. The editors of this issue did not know any of this when they invited me to do this review, but it was a major reason I accepted the invitation.

2. *We, as evaluation professionals, care about evaluation.* This entire issue epitomizes that caring. Stake could have been describing this issue of *New Directions for Evaluation* when he wrote: "We care about evaluation. We want to see others care about it. We want to encourage them to do it. We promote evaluation services, our own and those of our profession.

New Directions for Evaluation, no. 103, Fall 2004 © Wiley Periodicals, Inc.

163

We favor methods that evaluate well, and encourage others to use them too. It is an advocacy we flaunt" (2004, p. 104).

A powerful verb, *flaunt*. This volume *flaunts* the potential contribution of monitoring and evaluation (M&E) to solve the global HIV/AIDS crisis.

I count myself among those who care about evaluation generally and HIV/AIDS evaluation specifically. The experiences of those involved with the development and implementation of HIV/AIDS M&E systems provide us with a macrocosm of M&E more generally. The chapters in this issue represent much of what is good about evaluation—and also much of what is wrong with it. I would ask that my criticisms be understood in the context of caring about evaluation.

3. *"We advocate rationality."* The mindset of rationality constitutes a foundation that supports the M&E initiatives and recommendations that run throughout the chapters. Logic modeling is one common manifestation of rationality in evaluation, logic being a primary tool for rational thinking and a criterion against which we evaluate rationality. It is not surprising to learn, then, that the basic M&E organizing framework endorsed by all participating agencies is based on a simple "input-activities-output-outcome-impact" framework (Chapter Two, this issue).

Harkening back to the first advocacy in this list, however—that of caring about the thing being evaluated—I wonder whether we can find a place for *heart* and emotion amid all this heady stuff. Later in this review, I will rant (perhaps irrationally) on this concern.

4. *"We care to be heard. We are troubled if our studies are not used."* The M&E approaches described and analyzed in this issue are often labeled "utilization-focused M&E." That happens to be a matter of some interest to me as well as a little knowledge, so I will opine about the extent to which the M&E systems offered here manifest utilization-focused premises and, to the extent that they do, some of the dilemmas and challenges posed.

5. *"We are distressed by underprivilege. We see gaps among privileged patrons and managers and staff and underprivileged participants and communities."* In the global context, poverty and HIV/AIDS go hand in glove. Among the privileged are evaluators. The M&E systems described in this issue cost millions of dollars and provide privileged employment to thousands. Among other things, this raises the stakes to demonstrate that such expenditures, which directly reduce funds available for treating people afflicted with HIV/AIDS, ultimately add value and benefit underprivileged participants and communities. Whenever I conduct evaluation training in developing country settings, this question is always front and center. In this issue, as in most of evaluation, this nagging question of evaluation's ultimate cost-benefit remains one of hope and idealism rather than empirical demonstration.

6. *Finally, "We are advocates of a democratic society."* Operating in a global context of greatly diverse political systems, the efforts reported in this issue supersede variations in national political systems to accomplish

the goal of a universal and standardized HIV/AIDS M&E system around the world.

There is even evidence that dictators can be information users. De Lay and Manda open Chapter One by telling the story of how President Museveni of Uganda got his initial push to deal with HIV/AIDS from President Fidel Castro of Cuba, who called and told him that eighteen of the sixty Ugandan soldiers who had been sent for training in Cuba had tested positive for HIV. Uganda subsequently became one of the exemplar nations in turning back the tide of HIV/AIDS. Try mapping that outputs-to-outcomes-to-impacts logic model chain to explain and attribute high-impact information use.

Is HIV/AIDS M&E Different?

De Lay and Manda identify four ways in which the unique nature of HIV/AIDS may pose special challenges for M&E. First is global denial. De Lay and Manda argue that nation-states have handled HIV/AIDS differently from other infectious diseases. Prevalence numbers have been diminished, suppressed, or delayed and, when reported, explained away as being infections of foreigners. In short, it has been difficult to get governments to acknowledge the scale of the problem and to intervene in a timely manner, including supporting the collection of valid and reliable data about prevalence.

This is not, however, a problem specific to infectious diseases. Problems of child abuse, family and community violence, homelessness, mental illness, unemployment, rape, and corruption have suffered, and often still do, from underreporting, data manipulation, report suppression, and findings delay. Nor are these problems limited to developing countries.

Data used to monitor donor needs for program performance: I am afraid HIV/AIDS evaluations have no special claim here. As near as I can tell, it is a nearly universal phenomenon that the data most useful to local programs fail to provide what international donors want. Guess who wins in setting data priorities? Podems (2004) just completed a doctoral dissertation on this issue studying a youth program in South Africa. She offers a framework for attempting to improve communications between funders and local implementers using evaluation as a communications tool.

Protection of individual rights versus the public good: Tensions between the need for data and the right to privacy have emerged in a number of areas, although HIV/AIDS surely intensifies the stakes on both sides. But this tension is also manifest in trying to track child-support payments, sexual predators, genetic diseases, welfare fraud, unemployment benefits, foster care, adoptions, mental health, and family violence. One might say that there is almost an inherent tension between society's need to know to inform policy decisions and individuals' desire to protect themselves from government intrusion into their lives. Orwellian nightmares dominate this debate.

Selective application of evaluation research in support of ideologies and values: Selective use of evaluation data to support political bias, also worrisome to De Lay and Manda, and appropriately so, may actually be less in HIV/AIDS than in other areas. Public health has a long and distinguished tradition of getting the data out and getting findings out in a timely way. Yes, there are inevitably short-term efforts to manipulate data for political purposes in the public health area, but the stakes are typically so high and the professionalism of health staff so well established that these manipulations and distortions find their way into the public light, especially in the age of the Internet. No, HIV/AIDS has no special privilege here. The problem is simply widespread and endemic to politics.

Tensions Between Competing Purposes for Evaluation

M&E systems are asked to satisfy a number of competing purposes—for example, accountability, program improvement, management decision making, identifying effective models for dissemination, and supporting collaboration among partners. In Chapter Two, Rugg, Carael, Boerma, and Novak suggest that the primary purpose of the HIV/AIDS M&E system should ideally be program improvement. In reality, they found that donor reporting and accountability demands burden the system and engulf local data-collection efforts to such an extent that evaluation is little used for program improvement. This is one of the most common observations in evaluation. Accountability demands routinely trump hopes for and intentions of program improvement.

We see this tension in the chapters in this issue. Chapter Two emphasizes the program improvement uses of evaluation while acknowledging a need for accountability. Chapter Five, on developing and implementing M&E "in the new era of expanded care and treatment of HIV/AIDS," emphasizes accountability, with an occasional nod to program improvement. Emphasis matters.

In a similar vein, Wilson (Chapter Six) notes in his African capacity-building analysis that most M&E frameworks are not designed as management tools. This is related to the problem of trying to have the same system serve both accountability and program improvement purposes—a good idea in theory but one that seldom works in practice. These different purposes need different data and different analysis processes.

Another universal tension is between bottom-up and top-down design and utilization processes. Anie and Larbi (Chapter Eight) describe Ghana's approach as "bottom up." It is helpful to take local people through the process of understanding and accepting indicators developed by international experts, but that is not the same as a genuinely bottom-up process in which grassroots priorities set the agenda, determine the methods and process, and develop the indicators of choice. The language matters here as well. Calling something "bottom up" when it is not experienced that way locally can lead to later alienation and lack of use. One of the most common complaints I hear from people at the grassroots level is that they were told that a process was bottom-up when, in fact, the real agenda was acquiescence to a top-down design. Bringing the needs of national and international users together with the needs of local and regional users remains one of the great challenges of M&E. National stakeholders and their information needs typically trump local stakeholders and their information needs. It is not clear to me that that did not happen in Ghana, but I could be wrong. The point is that no evidence is offered that the process *was actually experienced* as bottom up.

To determine how use actually occurs at these different levels, we need more rigorous follow-up than is available here. Take the case of Thailand's experience, reported by Kanshana and others (Chapter Seven). To the authors' credit, substantial attention is given to M&E use. But what is offered falls short of telling readers how the results are actually used. For example:

> One of the important uses of this monitoring system is to provide data to indicate programmatic and geographical areas where coverage is not optimal so that national or local policies or practices can be adjusted to improve the program. To this end, program staff were trained on interpreting the nine standard reports; a series of regional and national meetings were held to bring together program staff and policymakers to review data, identify areas of successful and unsuccessful implementation, and identify solutions to improving the program.

So far, so good, but we are not told what actual program improvements were made, if any. The process sounds excellent, and the intentions are exquisitely utilization focused, but the unanswered question is whether anything important actually changed as a result of these meetings. Were the findings discussed actually used to make identifiably significant improvements to the program? A truly utilization-focused M&E system will include closing the loop by evaluating actual use and learning what factors enhanced use and what factors may have inhibited use, then using those learnings to further enhance use (Patton, 1997).

Humanizing M&E

I promised to return to advocacy of rationality and logic in evaluation, the third item on Stake's list. I wondered earlier whether we could find a place for heart and emotion in evaluation. Certainly I would not be so rash as to suggest a prominent place, but a place nonetheless. I was stimulated to ponder this question as a result of the overall impression I took from reading the contributions in this issue.

These chapters portray herculean efforts to create, organize, and implement rigorous and standardized M&E throughout the world. It is an ambitious, even staggering, undertaking. To get multiple and competing international agencies and jealous-of-their-autonomy governments around the world to agree to the "three ones" principle is an impressive achievement. One can only hope that this achievement lives up to its advance billing of better and more useful data. The danger and potential downside of perfectly coordinated and centralized data collection and reporting is that it can be harder to detect corruption and correct abuses. Monopolies require careful and transparent scrutiny and regulation. The three ones principle celebrates and institutionalizes an HIV/AIDS M&E monopoly. That may well yield important benefits of comparative data, efficiencies in data collection and analysis, and global economies of scale. It may also collapse under its own weight, which is my reading of the history of many such systems.

But I digress. The central point I want to make in this section is my overall impression of these HIV/AIDS M&E systems as highlighting numbers, reports, comparisons, collaborations, indicators—and systems. All of these things are important, indeed critical. But where are the portrayals of people living with HIV and dying of AIDS? I know, I know. That was not the purpose of this issue. But perhaps it should have been a purpose. Perhaps it should always be a purpose in evaluation to remind policymakers, journalists, diverse stakeholders, the general public, and evaluators that there are real people behind the numbers and data reports.

If I could wave a magic evaluation wand and change M&E evaluation reporting, it would be to mandate that monitoring data always be reported with stories about real people so that the numbers do not take on an abstract life of their own. These chapters portray millions of dollars being spent to create standardized systems and coordinated systems and performance systems and tracking systems and monitoring systems and data storage systems and data-sharing systems. Where are the people? Not just the people suffering from HIV/AIDS, although their absence from these chapters is a travesty, in my judgment. But I would also welcome stories about the people at the grassroots level who enter the data into these systems and those who are supposed to use these data. I have met many of these people in the workshops I do around the world. They offer a different perspective on global, standardized M&E systems. Evaluating those systems will ultimately need to include those stories and perspectives.

A Systems Perspective

Speaking of systems and perspectives, another overall impression I came away with from reading these chapters is how deeply entrenched mechanistic linearity is in evaluation. I do not share the authors' enthusiasm for the endorsement by all participating agencies of a simple input-activities-output-outcome-impact framework. This strikes me as an especially limited framework for understanding HIV/AIDS. The two cases of dramatic national reversal of HIV/AIDS infection rates with which I am most familiar, Uganda and Brazil, are fundamentally stories of complex, dynamic systems change. The stories differ in their specifics, but each involve multiple, overlapping interventions at different levels and in different ways to change national consciousness, community attitudes, cultural values, political priorities, and normative behaviors. Interdependent change occurred in religious communities, political policies, educational institutions, community organizing, public health, and criminal justice. Under such circumstances of massive, interconnected, and interdependent dynamic systems change across sectors, budgetary sources, and interventions (national, regional, and local), complex systems change mapping and networking models hold more promise than do traditional linear-logic models.

I had the opportunity to do evaluation training for a diverse group in South Africa. Participants included educators, health workers, police, environmentalists, park rangers, youth program staff, employment program managers, civil servants, and many others. All of them reported being involved in some way in the battle against HIV/AIDS infections regardless of their organization's mission. Firefighters, for example, were distributing HIV/AIDS information and supporting condom use. In such an environment, facing such a massive problem with such huge societal implications, the autonomous program may not be a meaningful unit of evaluation analysis. I certainly cannot imagine disentangling the various and overlapping interventions I have witnessed and heard about in various African countries. Yet, the dominant concept of evaluation in this issue is a traditional inquiry into an autonomous intervention delivered in a linear-outcomes model to isolate and attribute its impacts, including conducting quasi-experimental designs. I am openly skeptical about the utility of such designs in these circumstances. Indeed, the controls needed to even attempt such designs risk having the evaluation design interfere with the effective creation and implementation of complex and dynamic systems interventions that are too messy and emergent to be appropriately evaluated by static designs and linear, mechanistic attribution models.

Chapter Nine, on intervention research and program evaluation, epitomizes this limited perspective. Peersman and Rugg's four quality criteria for methodological rigor reflect the narrow view that, especially in dire circumstances where the stakes are high, evaluation is no different from research and must favor quantitative measures and linear, experimental attribution designs. These influential authors give token attention to alternative evaluation methods and none to complex systems dynamics.

In essence, I would argue that HIV/AIDS is best understood as a dynamic, complex systems phenomenon. To be useful and insightful, evaluation designs need to match the nature of the phenomenon. The evaluation framework celebrated in these chapters, while recommending that the simple linear approach be expanded to include the triangulation of data from multiple sources and methods, does not go far enough to embrace a systems framework and thus fails to map the nature of the phenomenon to the evaluation approach. In so saying, and in defense of the authors, I acknowledge that the M&E approaches presented here represent mainstream evaluation thinking, which is precisely the problem.

First Do No Harm

Evaluation is not benign. In addition to potentially wasting scarce resources and diverting desperately needed resources from treatment, evaluation can do harm in other ways. One of these is evaluating what are on the face of it unrealistic and overpromised goals, adding to the pretense that the goals are meaningful. Consider the "hard targets" of the United Nations General Assembly Special Session's Declaration of Commitment being adopted in national plans, as described in Chapter Three. Take just one example: "By 2005, ensure that at least 90 percent, and by 2010 at least 95 percent, of young men and women aged 15 to 24 have access to the information, education, including peer education and youth-specific HIV education, and services necessary to develop the life skills required to reduce their vulnerability to HIV infection, in full partnership with young persons, parents, families, educators, and health care providers."

This kind of goal guarantees failure. Where do such target outcomes come from? One of the common misperceptions about utilization-focused evaluation is that the evaluator simply yields passively to whatever stakeholders suggest, acquiescing to their perspective regardless of whatever absurdities they may offer. Quite the contrary, I have argued that every evaluation is a training opportunity to increase the sophistication of those involved, especially primary intended users, and that the evaluator has a stake in the integrity and sensibility of the evaluation. When goals are patently overpromised and unrealistic, based on generic evaluation knowledge about what is likely and possible, as is often the case and certainly the case for this goal, it becomes the evaluator's responsibility to facilitate careful consideration of the implications of proceeding. I reject the perspective that our job is simply to evaluate whatever goals we are handed without commentary on their sensibility and meaningfulness. *This is where we get to be advocates for rationality.*

A Microcosm of the Global Challenges

The authors of the chapters in this issue portray, on the whole, an unusual degree of success in creating and implementing a universally accepted M&E framework, including identification and standardization of key indicators. Those involved have also established standards for quality HIV/AIDS evaluations and have shown remarkable acumen in navigating the treacherous political and cultural shoals of HIV/AIDS to establish a global foundation for M&E. In this regard, these chapters, although focused on HIV/AIDS

M&E approaches, reflect the state of the art of evaluation more generally—the field's strengths, its shortcomings, and its controversies. I have offered some additional criteria for what constitutes success that calls into question some of the achievements touted in this issue.

The successes reported here in creating worldwide HIV/AIDS M&E systems also increase the stakes in making sure that the resulting findings are useful and actually used to reduce the infection rate, reduce deaths from AIDS, and assist those living with HIV/AIDS. Given the high costs of these systems, the stakes for evaluation are high. Can evaluators deliver on the promise that better information will lead to more effective policies and programs; better allocation of scarce resources; and better outcomes at local, national, and international levels? In that regard, the authors record and document important milestones in HIV/AIDS M&E globally. But the challenges ahead are at least as daunting as those already overcome, namely, demonstrating that monitoring data and evaluation findings are worth what they cost and can make a difference in the lives of people vulnerable to and afflicted by HIV/AIDS. Stay tuned. Given the visibility and importance of the global battle against HIV/AIDS, evaluation's contributions here are likely to ripple and affect perceptions about the value of M&E systems generally.

References

Patton, M. Q. *Utilization-Focused Evaluation*. (3rd ed.) Thousand Oaks, Calif.: Sage, 1997.

Podems, D. "Nonprofit Evaluation in South Africa: A Study of Relationships Between the Donor and Nonprofit Organizations in the Developing World." Unpublished doctoral dissertation, Union Institute and University, Cincinnati, 2004.

Stake, R. "How Far Dare an Evaluator Go Toward Saving the World?" *American Journal of Evaluation*, 2004, 25(1), 103–107.

MICHAEL QUINN PATTON is an International Consultant at the Union Institute and University in St. Paul, Minnesota.

INDEX